RAPID NURSING INTERVENTIONS:

Gerontologic

Delmar Publishers' Online Services
To access Delmar on the World Wide Web, point your browser to:
http://www.delmar.com/delmar.html
To access through Gopher:
gopher://gopher.delmar.com
(Delmar Online is part of "thomson.com," an Internet site with information on more than 30 publishers of the International Thomson Publishing organization.)
For more information on our products and services:
email: info@delmar.com or call 800-347-7707

RAPID NURSING INTERVENTIONS:

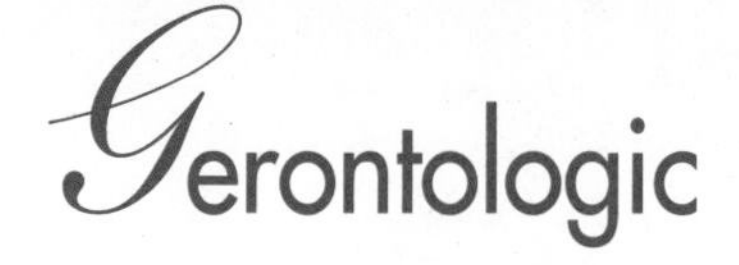

Ruth A. Mooney, BSN, MEd, MN, Ph.D.
Director, Clinical Practice and Research for Nursing
Philadelphia Geriatric Center
Philadelphia

Maryann M. Greenway, BSN, MSN, GNP, CS
Gerontologic Clinical Nurse Specialist
Philadelphia Geriatric Center
Philadelphia

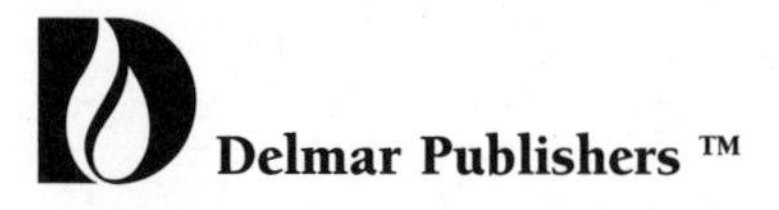

I(T)P™ An International Thomson Publishing Company

Albany • Bonn • Boston • Cincinnati • Detroit • London • Madrid
Melbourne • Mexico City • New York • Pacific Grove • Paris • San Francisco
Singapore • Tokyo • Toronto • Washington

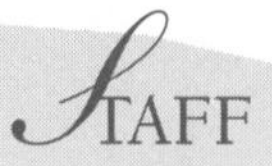

STAFF

Team Leader:
DIANE McOSCAR

Sponsoring Editors:
PATRICIA CASEY
BILL BURGOWER

Developed for Delmar Publishers by:
JENNINGS & KEEFE Media Development, Corte Madera, CA

Concept, Editorial, and Design Management:
THE WILLIAMS COMPANY, LTD., Collegeville, PA

Project Coordinator:
KATHLEEN LUCZAK

Editorial Administrator:
GABRIEL DAVIS

Production Editor:
BARBARA HODGSON

Manuscript written by:
TERRI A. GREENBERG

Text Design:
SHIRLEY EPPS ARTWORK, INC.

For information, address:
Delmar Publishers
3 Columbia Circle
Box 15015
Albany, NY 12212-5015

International Thomson Publishing Europe
Berkshire House 168-173
High Holborn
London, WC1V7AA
England

Thomas Nelson Australia
102 Dodds Street
South Melbourne, 3205
Victoria, Australia

Nelson Canada
1120 Birchmount Road
Scarborough, Ontario
Canada M1K 5G4

International Thomson Editores
Campos Eliseos 385, Piso 7
Col Polanco
11560 Mexico D F Mexico

International Thomson Publishing GmbH
Königswinterer Strasse 418
53227 Bonn
Germany

International Thomson Publishing Asia
221 Henderson Road
#05-10 Henderson Building
Singapore 0315

International Thomson Publishing Japan
Hirakawacho Kyowa Building, 3F
2-2-1 Hirakawacho
Chiyoda-ku, Tokyo 102
Japan

Printed in the United States of America

Published simultaneously in Canada by Nelson Canada, a division of The Thomson Corporation.

2 3 4 5 6 7 8 9 10 XXX 00 99 98 97 96

Library of Congress Cataloging-in-Publication Data
Mooney, Ruth, 1947-
Rapid nursing interventions: gerontologic/Ruth A. Mooney, Maryann M. Greenway.
p. cm. — (Rapid nursing interventions)
Includes bibliographical references and index.
ISBN 0-8273-7094-6
1. Geriatric nursing. I. Greenway, Maryann M., 1939-.
[DNLM: 1. Geriatric Nursing—methods—handbooks.
2. Nursing Process—handbooks. WY 49 M818r 1996]
RC954.M66 1996
610.73'65—dc20
DNLM/DLC
for Library of Congress 95-21869
CIP

TITLES IN THIS SERIES:

INSTANT NURSING ASSESSMENT:

- Cardiovascular
- Respiratory
- Neurologic
- Women's Health
- Gerontologic
- Mental Health
- Pediatric

RAPID NURSING INTERVENTIONS:

- Cardiovascular
- Respiratory
- Neurologic
- Women's Health
- Gerontologic
- Mental Health
- Pediatric

Suzanne K. Marnocha, RN, MSN, CCRN
Assistant Professor, College of Nursing
University of Wisconsin
Oshkosh, Wisconsin

Linda Moody, RN, FAAN, Ph.D.
Professor, Director of Research and Chair,
Gerontology Nursing
College of Nursing
University of South Florida
Tampa, Florida

Patricia A. O'Neill, RN, CCRN, MSN
Instructor, DeAnza College School of Nursing
Cupertino, California

Virgil Parsons, RN, DNSc, Ph.D.
Professor, School of Nursing
San Jose State University
San Jose, California

Elaine Rooney, MSN
Assistant Professor of Nursing, Nursing Department
University of Pittsburgh
Bradford, Pennsylvania

Barbara Shafner, RN, Ph.D.
Associate Professor, Department of Nursing
Otterbein College
Westerville, Ohio

Elaine Souder, RN, Ph.D.
Associate Professor, College of Nursing
University of Arkansas for Medical Sciences
Little Rock, Arkansas

Mary Tittle, RN, Ph.D.
Associate Professor, College of Nursing
University of South Florida
Tampa, Florida

Peggy L. Wros, RN, Ph.D.
Assistant Professor of Nursing
Linfield College School of Nursing
Portland, Oregon

Contents

NOTICE TO THE READER

The publisher, editors, advisors, and reviewers do not warrant or guarantee any of the products described herein nor have they performed any independent analysis in connection with any of the product information contained herein. The publisher, editors, advisors, and reviewers do not assume, and each expressly disclaims, any obligation to obtain and include information other than that provided to them by the manufacturer.

The reader is expressly warned to consider and adopt all safety precautions that might be indicated by the activities described herein and to avoid all potential hazards. By following the instructions contained herein, the reader willingly assumes all risks in connection with such instructions.

The publisher, editors, advisors, and reviewers make no representations or warranties of any kind, including but not limited to the warranties of fitness for particular purpose or merchantability, nor are any such representations implied with respect to the material set forth herein, and the publisher, editors, advisors, and reviewers take no responsibility with respect to such material. The publisher, editors, advisors, and reviewers shall not be liable for any special, consequential, or exemplary damages resulting, in whole or in part, from readers' use of, or reliance upon, this material.

A conscientious effort has been made to ensure that the drug information and recommended dosages in this book are accurate and in accord with accepted standards at the time of publication. However, pharmacology is a rapidly changing science, so readers are advised, before administering any drug, to check the package insert provided by the manufacturer for the recommended dose, for contraindications for administration, and for added warnings and precautions. This recommendation is especially important for new, infrequently used, or highly toxic drugs.

CPR standards are subject to frequent change due to ongoing research. The American Heart Association can verify changing CPR standards when applicable. Recommended Schedules for Immunization are also subject to frequent change. The American Academy of Pediatrics, Committee on Infectious Diseases can verify changing recommendations.

FOREWORD

As quality and cost effectiveness continue to drive rapid change within the health care system, you must respond quickly and surely—whether you are a student, novice, or expert. This Rapid Nursing Interventions series—and its companion Instant Nursing Assessment series—will help you do that by providing a great deal of nursing information in short, easy-to-read columns, charts, and boxes. This quick, convenient presentation will support you as you practice your science and art and apply the nursing process. I hope you'll come to look on these books as providing "an experienced nurse in your pocket."

The Rapid Nursing Interventions series is a handy source for step-by-step nursing actions to meet the fast-paced challenges of today's nursing profession. The Instant Nursing Assessment series offers immediate, relevant clinical information on the most important aspects of patient assessment. These books contain several helpful special features, including nurse alerts to warn you quickly about critical assessment findings, nursing diagnoses, charts that include interventions and rationales, along with collaborative management to help you work with your health-care colleagues, patient teaching tips, and the latest nursing research findings.

Each title in the Rapid Nursing Interventions series begins with a quick review of symptoms and focused assessment followed by the components of nursing intervention. From there, each book expands to cover the essential nursing interventions and rationales, collaborative management, outcomes, and evaluation criteria for important diagnoses covered in that title.

Both medical and nursing diagnoses are included to help you adapt to emerging critical pathways, care mapping, and decision trees. All these new guidelines help decrease length-of-stay and increase quality of care—all current health-care imperatives.

I'm confident that each small but powerful volume will prove indispensable in your nursing practice. Each book is formatted to help you quickly connect your assessment findings with the patient's pathophysiology—a cognitive connection that will further help you plan nursing interventions, both independent and collaborative, to care for your patients skillfully and completely. With the help and guidance provided by the books in this series, you will be able to thrive—and survive—in these changing times.

— Helene K. Nawrocki, RN, MSN, CNA
Executive Vice President
The Center for Nursing Excellence
Newtown, Pennsylvania
Adjunct Faculty, La Salle University
Philadelphia, Pennsylvania

SECTION I. SYMPTOMS AND INTERVENTION REVIEW

Chapter 1. Symptoms and Focused Assessment

▽ ▽ ▽ ▽ ▽ ▽ ▽

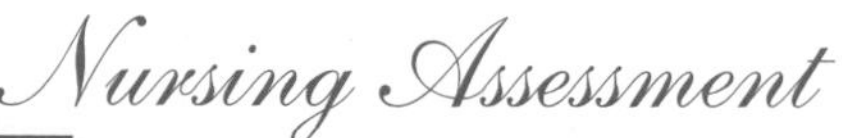

Nursing Assessment

SEE TEXT PAGES ______

Nursing assessment is the systematic, ongoing collection, verification, and communication of data about a particular patient from various sources throughout the care of the patient. It establishes a data base of information about a patient's level of wellness, health practices, past illnesses, and health care goals and needs.

Nursing assessment is the first step of the nursing process and influences the remaining steps: diagnosis, planning, implementation, and evaluation. The information collected during assessment provides the basis of an individualized plan of care for each patient.

Two types of data are collected during nursing assessment: subjective and objective.

- Subjective data, or symptoms, are the patient's perceptions about his or her health problems. Only the patient can provide this information. It usually includes feelings of anxiety, physical discomfort, and mental distress.
- Objective data, or signs, are the observations, perceptions, and measurements made by the nurse or other data collector. This information is usually obtained through physical examination, psychosocial assessment, clinical observations, and diagnostic studies.

Included in a patient's data base are the health history, physical assessment, psychosocial assessment, review of clinical records, and review of the literature.

Health History

The following information is included in the patient's health history.

- Biographic information—factual demographic data about the patient. Age, address, working status, marital status, and types of insurance are all important types of biographic information.
- Reasons for seeking health care—expressed and recorded in the patient's own words.
- Present illness or health concern—onset (sudden or gradual), duration, location, intensity, and quality of symptoms. Precipitating and alleviating factors also need to be assessed. It is appropriate to discuss the patient's and family's expectations of the health care team so that mutual and realistic goals can be established.
- Past health history—previous hospitalizations and surgeries; allergies to food, drugs, and pollutants, with specific reactions; alcohol, tobacco, caffeine, and drug use, including frequency and duration of use; nutritional habits; previous blood transfusions; and prescribed and self-prescribed medications.
- Family history—determination of risk factors for cancer, heart disease, diabetes mellitus, kidney disease, hypertension, and mental disorders. If any of the patient's immediate blood relatives have a history of a serious disease or are being treated for such a disease, details about the disease or condition, treatment, and response should be noted in the patient's record.
- Environmental history—exposure to pollutants and threats to physical safety.
- Psychosocial and cultural history—primary language, ethnic group, affect, coping skills, spiritual and social affiliations, and developmental stage.
- Review of systems—systematic approach to obtaining information about all body systems by questioning the patient about the normal functioning of each body system. Abnormalities are clearly and concisely documented.
- Self-care abilities—ability to bathe, feed, dress, and toilet himself or herself as well as ability to walk and potentially use walking aids (cane or walker).
- Discharge planning factors—destination after discharge; support systems, including family, friends, and community resources; and access to transportation, shopping, and health care facilities.

Physical Assessment

During a physical assessment, objective data are collected to verify or negate abnormalities, identify patient needs, and appropriately establish a plan of care.

The following are important things to remember when performing a physical assessment.

- Make clear, concise explanations to the patient about what you are doing, why you are doing it, and how long the examination will take.
- Assess what is appropriate for the patient's condition; establish priorities. For example, an elderly patient who fatigues easily may require minimal position changes, and a patient with chest pain may require only a quick cardiovascular assessment rather than a neurologic examination.
- Ensure the patient's privacy and provide good lighting and a quiet, restful environment.
- Carry out a systematic, thorough physical assessment to prevent omissions in data collection. The following are two examples of physical examination methods:
  - Head-to-toe approach—systematic assessment of the patient beginning at the head and ending at the toes
  - Body systems approach—systematic assessment of the patient according to a designated sequence of body systems
- Before proceeding with the examination, the nurse should make a general survey, which includes observation information related to mental status, body development, nutritional status, sex, race, chronologic versus apparent age, appearance, and speech.

The techniques used to perform a physical assessment include the following:

- Inspection—visualizing the patient's body. Visual inspection is combined with hearing and smelling. Inspection is often the best way to begin an examination because it is the assessment technique that is least threatening to the patient.
- Palpation—examining the surface of the body with light touch using the hands or fingers and examining the deeper body structures with deep palpation. This technique may be used to evaluate organ position, body temperature, abnormal growths, and abdominal rigidity as well as to identify the location of pain.
- Percussion—sharp tapping of the body surface to produce vibration of the underlying structures. This

technique is used to determine the position and size of organs and to check for the presence of fluid or air in a body cavity.
- Auscultation—listening with a stethoscope for heart, lung, and bowel sounds.

TECHNIQUE FOR APPLYING INDIRECT PERCUSSION

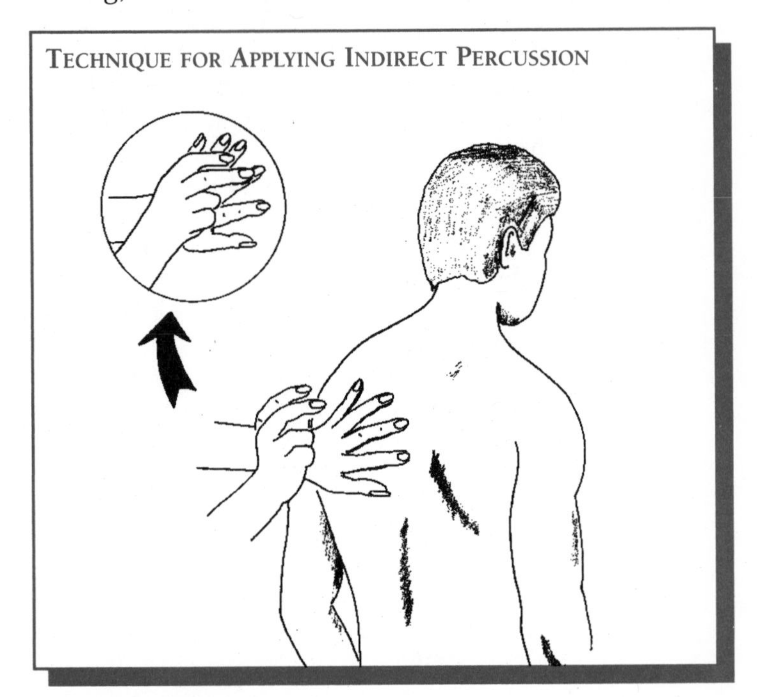

Psychosocial Assessment
- General appearance and behavior: includes motor ability, language ability, writing ability, and sensory function
- Sensorium: includes level of consciousness, orientation, attention span, memory, cognitive abilities, general knowledge, intellectual level, emotional state, and life situation
- Mental dysfunction, if present

Laboratory and Diagnostic Findings
Included in this data base component are baseline information, response to illness, and the effects of treatment methods.

The following are sources of data:
- *Interview with the patient.* The patient can usually provide the most accurate information regarding his or her health care needs, lifestyle patterns, past and present illnesses, and changes in activities of daily living. The patient interview requires effective communication tech-

niques, including interviewing skills and active listening. The nurse needs to be calm, unhurried, and relaxed. Ideally, the environment should be quiet and free from interruptions. To conclude the interview, the nurse should summarize the main points. The patient then has the opportunity to agree or disagree with the nurse's perceptions of his or her health problems.
- *Interview with the family.* Family members can be interviewed as primary sources of information when the patient is an infant or a child or is mentally handicapped, disoriented, or unconscious. The same techniques described for a patient interview apply to a family interview.
- *Consultation with other health care professionals.* This may include physicians, physical therapists, social workers, community health workers, and clergy. These people can provide information about how the patient interacts with the health care environment, reacts to results of diagnostic procedures, and responds to visitors. This consultation may also help the nurse to gather data about the social supports that are in place in the community so that effective discharge planning can be done.

Review of Clinical Records

This review verifies information about past health patterns and treatments or provides new information.

Review of the Literature

This review completes the data base by increasing the nurse's knowledge of appropriate treatments, symptoms, prognosis, and standards of therapeutic practice.

The last part of the assessment consists of the following processes:
- Validation of data by comparison with other sources, such as a comparison of subjective data with objective data
- Organization of information into meaningful clusters with focus on areas that need support and assistance for recovery

- Documentation of data, consisting of the recording of all observations collected during assessment. The documentation should be descriptive and concise and should not include the nurse's interpretations. The origins of descriptive data are in the patient's perception of the symptoms, the family's observations, the nurse's observations, and reports from other members of the health care team.

For example, a patient may describe chest pain as "an elephant sitting on my chest." The nurse's observations may be stated as follows:

"The patient clutches his chest with both hands. Patient keeps eyes tightly closed throughout assessment."

The nurse should not interpret the patient's behavior as "the patient tolerates pain poorly."

The nurse should report the information concisely, using correct medical terminology. For example, "Patient complains of substernal chest pressure radiating to the left arm, which began 2 hours ago related to moving the left arm. The pain has not been relieved with nitroglycerin, antacids, or rest."

From the recorded data, the nurse can formulate the appropriate nursing diagnoses.

Chapter 2. Nursing Interventions

▽ ▽ ▽ ▽ ▽ ▽ ▽

Outcome Development

Outcomes are descriptions of the behavior that a person will display if the care plan has been successful. They demonstrate resolution or reduction of the patient's problems as presented in the nursing diagnoses. Outcome statements need to be clear, concise, realistic, and patient-centered.

Nursing Interventions

Nursing interventions are actions directed toward assisting a patient to cope successfully with physical and emotional problems and to achieve the desired outcome. There are two types of nursing interventions: independent and collaborative.

- Independent interventions are treatments a nurse can prescribe and carry out without a physician's order. They do not require collaboration with other health care professionals. Assistance with activities of daily living (ADLs) related to hygiene is an independent nursing intervention. The scope of practice that a nurse can perform independently is licensed and mandated by the nurse practice act in the state in which the nurse works. Nurse practice acts vary from state to state.
- Collaborative interventions are shared with other health care team members. Many nursing interventions require an order from a physician. The nurse's role is to carry out the order and then assess the patient for desired or unfavorable outcomes. The nurse collaborates not only with the physician but also with other members of the health care team, such as dietitians, occupational therapists, physical therapists, dance therapists, music therapists, play therapists, and social workers.

Skills

To implement interventions, the nurse needs to demonstrate cognitive skills, interpersonal skills, and technical or psychomotor skills.

- Cognitive skills are the nurse's intellectual skills, such as problem solving, decision making, critical thinking, and innovation. The nurse needs to know the rationale for each intervention and to identify patient education and discharge needs. Cognitive skills are based on the nurse's education and experience. The nurse is responsible for the development of these cognitive skills through formal and informal educational opportunities.
- Interpersonal skills are the verbal and nonverbal communication skills that are used with the patient, family members, and health care team. The nurse must be able to communicate a concerned and caring attitude and to teach and counsel at a level compatible with the patient's understanding and emotional response.
- Technical or psychomotor skills are those used during implementation—for example, to prepare an injection, change a dressing, or manipulate equipment.

Implementation Methods

Assisting With ADLs

The nurse helps the patient perform activities and tasks that are performed in a normal day, such as bathing, dressing, and brushing teeth. The need for assistance with ADLs can be acute, chronic, temporary, permanent, or rehabilitative. For example, a postoperative patient may need assistance acutely for only 1 or 2 days after surgery. This is in contrast with a patient who has had a cerebrovascular accident and requires long-term, rehabilitative assistance. From the nursing assessment, the nurse can identify the amount of assistance needed for ADLs.

Counseling

The nurse helps the patient with problem solving and stress management by providing emotional, intellectual, spiritual, and psychological support. Counseling techniques used by the nurse promote a person's cognitive, behavioral, developmental, experiential, and emotional growth. They enable a patient to examine choices and thus gain a sense of control. To be effective, the nurse needs to develop a therapeutic relationship with the patient through the use of interpersonal skills.

Among the patients who need counseling are those who require lifestyle changes, such as smoking cessation, weight reduction, and decreasing activity levels. Also, patients who have chronic or disabling diseases need counseling to assist with the lifestyle changes and body image disturbances that they may encounter.

Patients and their families frequently need counseling when faced with death. The following counseling strategies are used by nurses:

- Behavior modification
- Bereavement counseling
- Biofeedback
- Relaxation training
- Reality orientation
- Crisis intervention
- Guided imagery
- Play therapy

Teaching

The nurse presents correct information about principles, procedures, and techniques to the patient. When providing education, the nurse must first assess the patient's learning needs, level of education, and motivation to learn.

Teaching and counseling are closely associated, in that they both involve communication skills to provide the patient with the tools needed to make a change. Teaching should be an ongoing process that builds on a person's knowledge base.

Performing Nursing Care Duties

The nurse needs to draw on his or her training and experience to perform specific care duties efficiently, smoothly, and accurately. These duties include the following:

- Evaluation and treatment of adverse reactions. An adverse reaction is a harmful or unintended effect of a medication or procedure. The nurse needs to know the potential undesired side effects to compensate for them, resulting in a reduction or an alleviation of the effects. For example, a nurse administering heparin should know that protamine sulfate will reverse the effects of heparin if bleeding problems result from its use.
- Preventive measures. Preventive nursing actions are aimed at preventing illness and promoting health.

Examples are assessment of the patient's health potential, health teaching, early diagnosis, and development of rehabilitation potential. The goal of preventive health measures is for the patient to achieve optimal wellness.
- Correct techniques in administering care and preparing a patient for procedures. The nurse needs knowledge and experience to carry out such procedures as changing dressings, inserting an indwelling catheter, and administering medications.
- Lifesaving measures. The purpose of a lifesaving measure is to restore physiologic or psychological stability, such as performing cardiopulmonary resuscitation, administering emergency medications, and restraining a violent patient. This type of intervention may be independent or collaborative.

Assisting the Patient to Attain Health Care Goals

The nurse adjusts care according to the patient's needs, stimulating and motivating the patient to achieve self-care and independence and encouraging the patient to accept care or follow the prescribed treatment regimen. In addition, the nurse and patient collaborate to achieve the goals they have developed together. Several methods can be used by the nurse to ensure that the patient achieves his or her goals.
- Provide the patient with enough privacy to meet basic needs but also be able to interact with the health care team. Orienting the patient to the health care facility fosters this independence and interaction.
- Provide for flexible, incremental, and attainable goals that the patient can successfully complete. With each level of independence a patient achieves, he or she goes on to the next level with more confidence in the ability to manage self-care requirements.
- Provide for adequate discharge planning and teaching to promote adherence to the treatment plan. The nurse needs to evaluate resources (personal and financial, for example) to promote a smooth transition to home.

For example, a cardiac patient with a two-story home may need a new home or some adjustments in his or her current home because of an inability to manage stairs. If this is not addressed before discharge, the patient may not adhere to the treatment plan. Counseling will help the patient and family make the changes needed because of the disease process or treatment.

Documentation

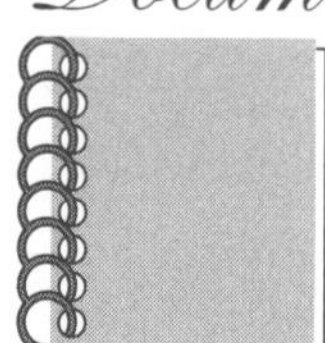

Documentation of nursing interventions is important for the following reasons:

- The patient's chart is a legal record of health care received.
- "If it is not recorded, it was not done."
- When a patient achieves his or her optimal level of wellness, the record shows the contribution that the nurse has made in this process.

It is important that the nurse document the following information objectively and concisely, using appropriate medical terminology:

- Date and time of the intervention
- Effectiveness of the intervention in achieving the proposed outcome
- Patient's progress toward resolution of the problem as stated in the nursing diagnosis

Suggested Readings

Ackerman, L. "Interventions Related to Neurologic Care." *Nursing Clinics of North America* 27, no.2 (1992): 325–347.

Brown, M. "How Do You Spell Assessment?...Simple Mnemonic Device to Organize Your Work." *American Journal of Nursing* 91 (September 1991): 55–56.

Bulechek, G. M., and J. C. McCloskey. "Defining and Validating Nursing Interventions." *Nursing Clinics of North America* 27, no. 2 (1992): 289–300.

Craft, M. J., and J. A. Willadsen. "Interventions Related to Family." *Nursing Clinics of North America* 27, no. 2 (1992): 517–540.

Hartman, D., and J. Knudson. "Documentation: A Nursing Data Base for Initial Patient Assessment." *Oncology Nursing Forum* 18 (January/February 1991): 125–130.

Hartrick, G., A. E. Lindsey, and M. Hills. "Family Nursing Assessment: Meeting the Challenge of Health Promotion." *Journal of Advanced Nursing* 20 (July 1994): 85–91.

Herr, K. A., and P. R. Mobily. "Interventions Related to Pain." *Nursing Clinics of North America* 27, no. 2 (1992): 347–371.

Loos, F., and J. Bell. "Circular Questions: A Family Interviewing Strategy." *Dimensions in Critical Care Nursing* 9, no. 1 (1990): 46–53.

Nelson, D. M. "Interventions Related to Respiratory Care." *Nursing Clinics of North America* 27, no. 2 (1992): 301–324.

Rakel, B. A. "Interventions Related to Patient Teaching." *Nursing Clinics of North America* 27, no. 2 (1992): 397–425.

Simons, M. R. "Interventions Related to Compliance." *Nursing Clinics of North America* 27, no. 2 (1992): 477–495.

Chapter 3. General Issues

▽ ▽ ▽ ▽ ▽ ▽ ▽

Introduction

Caring for the geriatric patient is a balancing act. Safety must be balanced against autonomy. Administration of medical therapy must be balanced against a patient's right to noncompliance. The treatment of one disorder or condition must be balanced against the treatment of another disorder or condition. The need to preserve the patient's functional abilities must be balanced against the need for expediency in treatment.

Sometimes we forget that geriatric patients are first and foremost people and not just assortments of symptoms and risk factors. Various factors contribute to an elderly patient's loss of personal identity.

- Many times the patient's family and caregivers place little value on the patient as a person, perhaps reflecting society's opinions.
- The same bureaucratic structure that ensures adequate treatment for all patients can also fail to view patients as individuals. Modern record-keeping technology has reduced the patient to just another number. A patient often thinks that everyone shares that opinion.
- In an effort to provide consistent service and care and meet cost-efficiency goals, sometimes personalized attention is sacrificed.

Symptom Range and Interactions

It's important to remember that for your patient, the important thing is his or her symptoms. Although trends can describe the conditions, diseases, and disorders that are common in the geriatric population, your patient has his or her own personal configuration of symptoms.

The interactions between one symptom and another, between symptoms and lifestyle choices, and between symptoms and the patient's overall health and condition are also unique to an individual patient.

Certainly, your assessments and interventions do not take place in a vacuum. An understanding of the patterns that research has discovered in geriatric health will help you to determine the correct course of treatment. Remember, however, that ultimately, you will have to manage this patient's symptoms to promote and ensure adequate care and a high quality of life.

Myths About Aging

Some assumptions can be detrimental to assessment of and interventions for the geriatric patient. Forgetting to consider the individual is certainly one of them.

Myth 1: Aging is a pathologic condition. Aging, in and of itself, is not a disease or an illness. It may bring greater risks to the patient suffering from a disease or an illness, but it's not something a patient recovers from. If, as a caregiver, you believe that there is something inherently negative about growing older, there's a good chance you will pass that impression along to your patients.

Caregiver attitude plays an important role in how a patient thinks of himself or herself. You must be diligent in maintaining a positive attitude toward an aging patient. When planning care and completing interventions, focus on treating the illness or condition and have as your goal the restoration of as much functionality as possible to the patient. Emphasize the need to "use it or lose it." Explain that continued exercise, mental stimulation, and social interaction help to prevent functional decline.

Myth 2: Confusion is a natural consequence of growing older. In a related manner, many people assume that mental acuity dulls with age. Confusion, dementia, and delirium represent serious risks to your patient and should be immediately evaluated and treated.

To assume that "Nana just isn't with it anymore" is to overlook symptoms of potentially fatal conditions, such as infection or a neurologic disorder.

The fact that dementia can underlie an episode of delirium must also be taken into account. Each condition can mask symptoms of the other. In addition, your patient may suffer from depression, which can increase the complexity of assessment and intervention.

Myth 3: Incontinence is an irreversible condition. This assumption ignores the way in which multiple symptoms can overlap, making assessment and intervention difficult. Maintaining continence is a vital element of maintaining self-esteem. In fact, incontinence is a primary reason for nursing home placement.

Careful assessment of all factors involved in a person's continence problems is the first step toward finding a solution. Eliminating or reducing the impact of each factor can go a long way toward restoring this important aspect of a person's functionality.

Myth 4: Older people don't abuse drugs. Substance abuse is not limited to younger patients. Geriatric patients have access to the same substances as younger patients: alcohol, illicit drugs, and marijuana.

If you neglect to evaluate your patient for signs of abuse, you may ignore a potentially fatal risk factor.

Certainly, if routine medication usage can cause serious adverse effects for your patient, adding uncontrolled drugs of unknown dose and potency can complicate the picture. Besides evaluating your patient for the use of illicit substances and alcohol, also be on the lookout for abuse of over-the-counter preparations, such as sedatives and laxatives. These medications can cause problems when used to excess or when combined with other drugs.

Delirium, dementia, and depression are also made worse by the addition of substance abuse.

Myth 5: Sexuality declines as one grows older. Many of your patients may share this opinion, but many more certainly do not. Various issues surrounding sexuality may be of concern to your patient, including the following:

- Effects of illness, medication, altered functionality, or other conditions on the patient's sexuality
- Normal course of changes the menopausal woman may experience
- Expression and fulfillment of sexual needs at a time when society expects these desires to be absent or diminished
- Inappropriate sexual behavior, such as behavior that might be displayed by a patient suffering from dementia

Some geriatric patients find it difficult to express their thoughts, concerns, and questions about their sexuality. Encourage your patient to take his or her time. Don't rush the person into a discussion if the time is not right. Respect the patient's desire for privacy and dignity. Provide information in a variety of formats—for example, written information or videotapes.

Encourage your patient to view expressions of sexuality as a natural part of life. Be sure to educate the patient about such important issues as safer sex, contraception (if required), and the effects of life cycle changes.

Caregiver Stress

Your patient does not live in isolation. Many people are involved in his or her care, whether the patient lives in a nursing home, an assisted-care facility, or his or her own home.

Arrangements for care are as varied as the patients you treat. Some patients manage most of their own care. Some are cared for by family or other "volunteer" caregivers. Still others employ aides with a range of skill levels. Nursing homes provide care environments for other patients.

In each case, other people are involved. These people have concerns of their own: health, financial, social, emotional, professional. When the responsibility for caring for your patient is added to the workload, the caregiver can experience caregiver stress or burnout.

The Older Caregiver

If your patient is being cared for by someone of similar age, such as a spouse or other domestic partner, a sibling, or a companion, that caregiver may be experiencing many of the same problems as the patient. Sometimes the choice of caregiver varies, depending on which person is currently feeling better than the other.

The Younger Caregiver

Much publicity has been focused on members of the "sandwich" generation. These caregivers often manage the responsibility of caring for their children and partners as well as caring for older relatives, such as their parents.

Sandwiched between these two generations, these caregivers experience stress related to the need to be in at least two places at once, the need to provide quality care for their families, and the resentment and guilt generated by their having to care for their parents.

Indications of Caregiver Stress

Circumstances that in one family may cause severe caregiver stress are easily managed in another family. The following are some indications that the caregiver is at risk for burnout:

- The caregiver himself or herself suffers from chronic disease or pain, impaired functionality, or dementia.
- The caregiver is solely (or largely) responsible for all patient care activities.
- The caregiver is responsible for the patient's care as well as his or her own family's care.
- The caregiver has a history of substance abuse, violence, or psychiatric disorders. In this case, caregiver stress may result in abuse of your patient.
- The caregiver is caring for a person with multiple self-care deficits who requires attention in many areas.

Intervening to Reduce or Eliminate Caregiver Stress

You may be alerted to possible caregiver stress by a report from the patient or by your assessment of the patient's condition. Or you may discover clues when talking with the caregiver. The caregiver may also specifically report problems with the responsibilities he or she bears.

Once the issue has been brought out into the open, discuss the causes and potential solutions with the caregiver.

The caregiver may be able to manage successfully most of the time. At other times or under certain circumstances, stressors arise that provoke feelings of being overwhelmed, such as the following:

- Insufficient time to accomplish caretaking activities
- Inadequate knowledge of patient care
- Emotional demands from the patient
- Conflicting demands from the patient and other important members of the family
- Financial concerns

Each caregiver must find his or her own methods for coping with the situation. The most effective methods may be a combination of techniques the caregiver has previously used to ease stress and newly developed strategies that you may suggest, such as the following:
- Asking for assistance from other family members
- Cutting back on additional commitments
- Setting more realistic goals
- Taking time for himself or herself

Once the caregiver has identified potential solutions, help him or her find ways to use these measures to cope with the stressors that are causing burnout.

Suggest additional resources that may be unknown to the caregiver, such as the following:
- Support groups
- Home health care aid
- Educational programs
- Caregiver respite programs
- Elder day-care centers

Your goal in intervening in cases of caregiver stress should be to find ways to help restore the caregiver's emotional equilibrium. Listen to the caregiver's concerns and complaints in a nonjudgmental way. When appropriate, suggest ways to alleviate the problems.

NURSE ALERT:
Caregiver stress is a significant risk factor in elder abuse. In fact, the profile of the most common abuser indicates that she is the daughter of the patient in whose home the patient lives.

Selected Resources for the Geriatric Patient or Caregiver

American Association of Retired Persons
1909 K Street
Washington, DC 20005
202-872-4700

Alzheimer's Disease and Related Disorders Association, Inc.
919 North Michigan Avenue
Suite 1000
Chicago, IL 60611
800-272-3900

Gray Panthers
2025 Pennsylvania Avenue NW
Suite 821
Washington, DC 20006
202-466-3132

National Aging Resource Center on Elder Abuse
810 First Street NE
Suite 500
Washington, DC 20002
202-682-2470

National Association for Home Care
519 C Street, NE
Washington, DC 20002
202-547-6157

National Council on Aging
409 Third Street SW
Washington, DC 20024
202-479-1200

National Institute of Aging
National Institutes of Health
Bethesda, MD
301-496-4000

Social Security Administration
Office of Public Inquiries
6401 Security Boulevard
Baltimore, MD 21235

Nursing Home Information Service
National Council of Senior Citizens
925 15th Street NW
Washington, DC 20005
202-347-8800

Chapter 4. Symptom Management

▽ ▽ ▽ ▽ ▽ ▽ ▽

Introduction

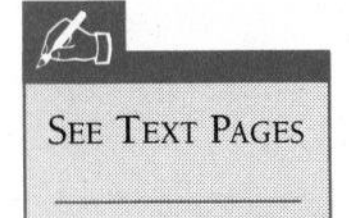

SEE TEXT PAGES ________

Sometimes investigating the health complaints of your geriatric patient may be comparable to searching for the proverbial needle in a haystack. Symptoms overlay symptoms. The patient may present with one set of symptoms on one day and with an entirely new set on the next day. Symptoms may fluctuate in severity and frequency.

Signs and symptoms of common disorders may mimic normal aging changes or be absent altogether. For example, your elderly patient may not experience the chest pain that is commonly associated with myocardial infarction.

One of your roles is to help sort through the bewildering array of complaints, history, physical findings, and test results to find a pattern. Once this pattern is tentatively identified, the health care team can begin interventions and treatment.

Information logs are a good way to begin to piece together a pattern. Symptom logs are one kind of information log. Medication and dietary logs are other kinds.

Logging information about problems at the time of occurrence helps to address the following problems:

- Inconsistent memory. Your patient may remember a fall and describe it in great detail, only for you to discover later that the incident was exaggerated. It's just as likely that the patient may not even remember the incident.
- Lack of causative factors. Describing a behavior problem, for example, requires not only narration of the patient's actions but narration of any precipitating event as well. If the description is made soon after the event, the supporting details will still be fresh in the mind.
- Witness availability. Sometimes other people's input is important to the accuracy of the report. Asking for input quickly eliminates the need to track down those people later.

Important Logs

There are several types of information logs that can be kept to help monitor the patient's care.

Continence Log

A continence log, also called a bladder diary or voiding log, can provide information that is useful in managing treatment of many varieties of incontinence. It can, for example, help the patient in bladder retraining or provide information for the nursing home staff about the patient's normal voiding pattern to help avoid accidents.

Information is usually recorded on a daily basis in the continence log and includes the following:

- Amount of fluid consumed
- Time of each toileting incident
- Description of the toileting incident
  - Used the toilet
  - Slight accident
  - Major accident
- Reason for an accident, if known, such as:
  - Delay in reaching toilet
  - Strong urge
- Record of pelvic exercises, if the patient is required to perform them

If the patient is in a nursing home setting, the following additional information will be helpful to the staff:

- Level of mobility
- Level of assistance required
- Preferred toileting pattern
  - Sitting or standing
  - Commode, urinal, toilet
- Medications that may alter continence patterns
- Infection, constipation, or other conditions that may alter continence patterns
- Involvement in a urinary continence program
- Effective strategies to encourage continence if the patient is resistive to toileting

Risk Assessment for Falls

Identifying the patient who is at risk for falls can help eliminate the occurrence of falls or near falls. Assessment of a patient's risk for falling should be part of the routine evaluation. The assessment should be brought up to date on a regular schedule and with every major change the patient experiences, such as new medications, illness, or injury.

Information that identifies the patient's risk for falling includes the following:

- History of previous falls or near falls
- History of dizziness or syncope
- Gait or balance disturbance
- Mental state disturbance, such as delirium or dementia
- History of seizures
- Decreased mobility
- Use of medications such as:
  - Antipsychotics
  - Antidepressants
  - Antiparkinsonian drugs
  - Antianxiety medications
  - Antihistamines
  - Antinauseants
  - Antidiarrheals
  - Antisecretory agents
  - Anti-inflammatories
  - Antihypertensives
  - Antianginals
  - Antiarrhythmia agents
  - Anticonvulsants
  - Narcotic analgesics
- Impaired sensory perception
  - Vision
  - Hearing
  - Touch
  - Proprioception
- Illness or other condition that may cause falls, alter balance, or decrease motor skills, as in the neurologic disorder Parkinson's disease

Activities of Daily Living Scales

Accurately measuring a patient's ability to complete activities of daily living (ADLs) is crucial to providing appropriate care while promoting patient autonomy. Each patient should be encouraged to complete as much of the self-care task as possible.

ADL scales include information about the following:
- Bathing
- Grooming
- Toileting
- Dressing
- Mobility
- Eating

Instrumental Activities of Daily Living Scales

Additional information may be included in your assessment to describe instrumental activities of daily living (IADLs), such as the following:
- Ability to complete financial transactions
- Ability to complete home repairs and maintenance
- Ability to shop for food

IADLs are those self-maintenance activities that are not directly related to personal care but are important in maintaining independent living.

Sample Assessment Chart

A sample assessment chart with categories describing ADLs and IADLs, along with selected physical attributes, appears on the following pages. Your institution may use a similar form.

Rehabilitation Care Assessment

		D	E	N
COGNITIVE	Short-term memory			
0 = No impairment	Long-term memory			
1 = Impairment	Decision making			
COMMUNICATION	Makes needs known			
PHYSICAL FUNCTION	Bed mobility			
I = Independent	Transfer			
S = Supervision	Locomotion			
A1 = Assist of 1	Dressing			
A2 = Assist of 2	Eating			
	Toileting			
	Personal hygiene			
	Bathing			
NURSING REHAB	Range of motion			
x If present	Splint/brace			
	Locomotion/ambulatory			
	Locomotion/wheel chair			
	Transfer			
	Dressing			
	Grooming			
	Bathing			
	Bladder training			
	Amputation care			
	Dining			
	Reorientation			
CONTINENCE	Bowel			
C = Continent	Bladder			
I = Incontinent	Diapers			
PSYCHOLOGICAL	Express of distress			
x If present	Wakes early/unpleasant			
	Sad/anxious mood			
	Motor agitation			
	Fails to eat/take medications			
	Withdrawal			
	Thoughts of death			

D = Days E = Evenings N = Nights

		D	E	N
BEHAVIOR	Wandering			
x If present	Verbally abusive			
	Physically abusive			
	Socially inappropriate			
	Hallucinations			
	Resists care			
	Physical restraints			
	Behavior mgmt program			
HEALTH COND	Urinary tract infection			
x If present	Pain			
	Fever			
	Vomiting			
	Diarrhea/constipation			
	Pneumonia			
	Aspiration			
	Falls			
	Seizures			
SKIN CONDITION	Stasis ulcer			
x If present	Pressure ulcer			
	Open lesion			
OTHER	Foley catheter			
x If present	Ostomy			
	Supplement			
	Tube feeding			
ASSISTIVE DEVICE				
Write in assistive device				
for eating in spaces to				
the right				
THERAPY	Respiratory			
Days/wk	Physical			
	Occupational			
	Speech			
	Psychology			

Source: Adapted from a form developed by the Nursing Documentation Commitee, Philadelphia Geriatric Center.

Behavioral Logs

Patient behavior, especially catastrophic episodes, pose several challenges to the patient care provider. If the behaviors are violent, the patient may harm himself or herself, other patients, or the caregiver. Discovering patterns in behavior can help to prevent episodes of negative behavior.

When recording information about patient behavior, include the following information:

- Time of day
- Location
- Activity (such as mealtime, bathing, dressing)
- Description of the behavior (such as striking out, verbal expressions, resistance to care)
- Precipitating factors, if identifiable
- Changes from routine (new staff member, deviation from regular schedule)
- Change in physical condition
- Change in medication
- Interventions taken to reduce the effect of the behavior
- Medications given specifically for the negative behavior
- Results of interventions

DAILY BEHAVIOR CHECKLIST

Philadelphia
Geriatric Center ______________________________

INITIALS	SIGNATURE	INITIALS	SIGNATURE	INITIALS	SIGNATURE

PROBLEM BEHAVIOR ______________________________ PATIENT'S NAME

7-3																														
3-11																														
11-7																														

						COMMENTS:
7-3						
3-11						
11-7						

PROBLEM BEHAVIOR ______________________________ PATIENT'S NAME

						COMMENTS:
7-3						
3-11						
11-7						

FILL IN DATE ON TOP ROW OF THE COLUMN. PLACE YOUR INITIALS IN THE BOX BELOW THE DATE IF THE BEHAVIOR HAS OCCURRED. IF THE BEHAVIOR HAS NOT OCCURRED, PLACE YOUR INITIALS IN THE BOX BELOW THE DATE *AND CIRCLE YOUR INITIALS*. WRITE COMMENTS AS NEEDED

Source: Developed by the Nursing Documentation Committee, Philadelphia Geriatric Center.

Medication Inventory

Polypharmacy is a major concern in caring for the geriatric patient. One of the best methods for conducting a medication inventory is to have the patient or caregiver bring all medications the patient is taking—both prescription and over-the-counter—to review.

Examine each medication, and ask the patient or caregiver to identify the following information about each product:
- Name
- Purpose
- Dose
- Schedule
- Special instructions
- Danger signs
- Length of time the patient has been using the product
- Food-related precautions
- Effects the drug has on the patient

Be sure to ask about the patient's use of caffeine, alcohol, and nicotine when completing the inventory.

The medication inventory should be completed regularly to ensure that the patient has not made any adjustments to the regimen, such as adding an over-the-counter drug. Regular inventories also help to prevent medication hoarding, determine if the entire course of medication was completed, and eliminate out-of-date medications.

Balancing Safety and Autonomy

Sometimes it may seem to your patient that "big brother" is indeed watching. Completing survey after survey and being asked to answer questions about subjects the patient considers private are taxing to everyone, not just the geriatric patient.

When working to complete an information log, keep in mind that your patient deserves privacy and respect. This may lead to a delay in getting all the information you require.

As with every other aspect of geriatric care, gathering information is a balancing act. Having the right information at the right time may help the patient to escape serious injury.

Reporting Accuracy

One last element to consider when collecting information about your patient is the accuracy of the data. You may have reason to believe that some information is inaccurate, poorly remembered, exaggerated, or omitted.

If possible, the best source of information is your firsthand experience. However, consider other sources of information about the patient, such as the following:
- Family members
- Companions
- Other caregivers

Your patient's confidence should be respected to the highest degree possible. You may, however, encounter situations in which you need independent confirmation of information the patient has reported to you.

Suggested Readings

Haight, Barbara, ed. "The Challenge of Caring: Behavioral Management." *Journal of Gerontological Nursing* 18 (1992): 39–40.

Hogstel, Mildred O., ed. *Nursing Care of the Older Adult.* Albany, NY: Delmar Publishers, 1994.

Kopac, Catherine A., ed. *Gerontological Nursing Certification Review Guide for the Generalist, Clinical Specialist, and Nurse Practitioner.* Potomac, MD: Health Leadership Associates, 1993.

Needham, Joan F. *Gerontological Nursing: A Restorative Approach*. Albany, NY: Delmar Publishers, 1993.

Trunk, Sandra, Elizabeth M. Tomquist, Mary T. Champagne, and Ruth A. Wiesel, eds. *Key Aspects of Elder Care: Managing Falls, Incontinence, and Cognitive Impairment*. New York: Springer Publishers, 1992.

Chapter 5. Falls

▽ ▽ ▽ ▽ ▽ ▽ ▽

Introduction

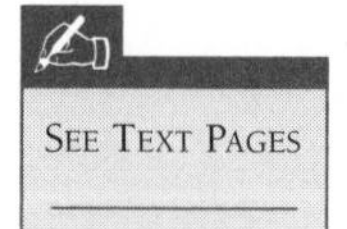

Falling poses a serious health hazard to geriatric patients. Studies conducted to determine the risk factors, rates of injury and morbidity, and economic impact involved in falling reveal the following results:

- Each year, about 9,500 persons over age 65 die as a result of falling, making it the number one cause of accidental death in this age-group.
- Falling is the most common accident in the home.
- Falls pose a greater risk to hospitalized elderly patients than to any other hospitalized population.
- Thirty percent to 50% of nursing home residents experience falls annually.
- One percent to 5% of falls result in fractures; 5% to 10% result in severe soft tissue injury.
- The primary reason for the use of patient restraint in nursing home settings is to prevent falls, even though research consistently demonstrates that restraints do not prevent falls.

The physical injuries caused by falls and near falls are only part of the clinical picture. Health care professionals must also be aware of the effects of falling on patient confidence, self-esteem, and autonomy.

By far, the most effective interventions involve prevention of falls by establishing a safe environment, increasing patient functionality, and supporting patient autonomy.

Identifying the Patient at Risk

Many factors come into play when a patient falls. Environmental factors can complicate impaired sensory function, for example. For this reason, there is no definitive picture of the patient at risk. There are many common characteristics, however, and each patient should be evaluated for his or her individual risk.

Risk factors associated with falls include the following:

- Previous incidents of falling
- Environmental factors
  - Poor lighting
  - Slippery surfaces
  - Loose floor covering, especially throw rugs
  - Obstructed pathways
  - Unstable, malfunctioning, or unfamiliar furniture
  - Improper footwear
- Physiologic factors
  - Impaired vision
  - Poor muscle tone
  - Impaired sense of balance
  - Gait disturbances
  - Blood pressure changes, especially orthostatic and postprandial blood pressure drop
  - Impaired hearing
  - Decreased tactile or kinesthetic senses
  - Porous bones
- Pathologic factors
  - Adverse drug reactions
  - Effects of surgery
  - Acute illness
  - Inadequate nutrition or hydration
  - Mental status disturbance, such as delirium or dementia
- Other factors
  - Use of physical or chemical restraints
  - Social isolation
  - Substance abuse
  - Reduced financial resources, preventing needed alterations and repairs

NURSING DIAGNOSIS: HIGH RISK FOR INJURY

RELATED TO:

- *Diminished sense of sight, hearing, touch, motion, or balance*

Nursing Interventions	Rationales
• Increase ambient lighting, especially in and around stairwells and corners.	• To decrease shadows and other vision-impairing effects
• Reduce the use of heavily patterned floor covering.	• To lessen the possibility of disorientation

Nursing Interventions *(continued)*	Rationales *(continued)*
• Provide a nightlight in the bedroom and bathroom or a flashlight for use if the patient gets up during the night.	• To reduce the risk that the patient will attempt to traverse rooms and hallways in the dark
• Provide easily seen visible signals, such as contrasting paint strips on stairs, or physical signals, such as handles or knobs at the top and bottom of staircases, to alert the patient to dangerous areas.	• To increase the likelihood that the patient will perceive the area that requires greater care to navigate
• Reduce the amount of clutter or extraneous equipment in the patient's environment.	• To avoid confusing the patient or presenting too many obstacles for the patient to navigate safely
• Locate the patient's eyeglasses and other frequently used items within easy reach.	• To discourage the patient from attempting to walk about without glasses or in search of the commonly needed items
• Avoid changing the layout or location of the patient's room.	• To reduce patient confusion
• Reduce traffic and confusion in halls and other common passageways.	• To minimize patient confusion and environmental press as risks of falling

COLLABORATIVE MANAGEMENT

Interventions	Rationales
• Consult with vision, hearing, and other specialists about devices that can increase patient functionality.	• To improve awareness of the environment, decrease confusion, and decrease the risk of falling.

NURSING DIAGNOSIS: HIGH RISK FOR INJURY (*continued*)

OUTCOME:	EVALUATION CRITERIA:
• The patient will be free from injury and able to function to the best of his or her abilities.	• There is no report or evidence of physical injury. • There is no report of falls.

NURSING DIAGNOSIS: HIGH RISK FOR INJURY

RELATED TO:

- *Use or abuse of medications, both prescribed and over-the-counter*

Nursing Interventions	Rationales
• Monitor the patient's medications: dose, frequency, purpose, actual use, and compliance.	• To identify medication that may contribute to a fall, either by itself or in combination with other medications
• Instruct the patient in the proper use of the medications he or she must take.	• To reduce the possibility of misuse that could contribute to a fall
• When assessing a patient who has fallen, be sure to ask about recent use of medication.	• To determine if the medication could have been a factor in the fall

COLLABORATIVE MANAGEMENT

Interventions	Rationales
• Consult with the health care provider concerning alternative medications or dosage schedules, if appropriate.	• To provide the patient with effective therapy while reducing the risk of falling

OUTCOME:	EVALUATION CRITERIA:
• The patient will be free from injury and able to function to the best of his or her abilities.	• There is no report or evidence of physical injury. • There is no report or evidence of falls.

NURSING DIAGNOSIS: HIGH RISK FOR INJURY

RELATED TO:

- *Elimination needs or need for food or drink*

Nursing Interventions	Rationales
• Anticipate the patient's needs for toileting, eating, or drinking.	• To prevent injury if the patient attempts to fulfill these needs by himself or herself
• Respond quickly to patient requests.	• To reduce the possibility of the patient's attempting to complete the task alone
• Explain to the patient, using appropriate language, the limits on his or her mobility.	• To help the patient understand when to ask for help
• Lower the bed or side rails.	• To make it easier for the patient to get up from the bed when necessary and to reduce the potential for serious injury if the patient does fall

NURSE ALERT:
Research has shown that the use of restraints actually increases the danger associated with falls.

Nursing Interventions	Rationales
• Provide a bedside commode or urinal, if appropriate.	• To make toileting more convenient and safer for the patient
• Make sure the patient's belongings are within easy reach.	• To eliminate the need for the patient to move about to retrieve them

COLLABORATIVE MANAGEMENT

Interventions	Rationales
• Discuss specific patient needs with the health care team to determine his or her needs, strengths, and limitations.	• To reduce the risk of falls while promoting maximum independence and functionality.

NURSING DIAGNOSIS: HIGH RISK FOR INJURY *(CONTINUED)*

OUTCOME:	EVALUATION CRITERIA:
• The patient will be free from injury and able to function to the best of his or her abilities.	• There is no report or evidence of physical injury. • There is no report or evidence of falls.

NURSING DIAGNOSIS: HIGH RISK FOR INJURY

RELATED TO:

- *General weakness or weakness caused by recent surgery or illness*

Nursing Interventions	Rationales
• Establish a routine for toileting, meals, exercise, and social activities.	• To reduce patient isolation and reassure the patient that his or her needs will be met
• Encourage the patient to ambulate within his or her best ability, with assistance as needed.	• To reduce the possibility of muscle atrophy from disuse
• Encourage the patient to complete some exercise, if possible. If the patient cannot complete exercises independently, assist him or her to complete range-of-motion exercises.	• To restore muscle function, prevent contractures, or prevent or slow decline

COLLABORATIVE MANAGEMENT

Interventions	Rationales
• Consult with physical or occupational therapy staff for exercises the patient can do to improve muscle tone and strength or about assistive devices the patient can use.	• To improve patient functionality

NURSING DIAGNOSIS: HIGH RISK FOR INJURY *(CONTINUED)*

OUTCOME:	EVALUATION CRITERIA:
• The patient will be free from injury and able to function to the best of his or her abilities.	• There is no report or evidence of physical injury. • There is no report or evidence of falls.

NURSING DIAGNOSIS: HIGH RISK FOR INJURY

RELATED TO:

- *Cognitive impairment*

Nursing Interventions	Rationales
• Provide a nightlight in the bedroom and bathroom.	• To reduce the risk that the patient will misinterpret areas of shadow and not recognize the bathroom
• Answer patient requests for assistance promptly.	• To reduce the possibility of the patient's attempting to get out of bed unaided and wandering
• Use a motion-sensitive bed alarm to identify patient attempts to get out of bed unaided.	• To reduce the possibility of the patient's attempting to get out of bed unaided and wandering
• Position the bed at its lowest level, with the side rails lowered.	• To reduce the risk of injury if the patient should climb or fall out of bed
• Encourage the patient to go to the toilet at regular intervals throughout the night.	• To reduce the risk of injury from an unassisted attempt to get out of bed and walk to the bathroom

COLLABORATIVE MANAGEMENT

Interventions	Rationales
• Engage the staff in providing meaningful activities for the patient throughout the day.	• To provide a focus for the patient's activities and reduce agitation, which is a risk factor for increased falls

NURSING DIAGNOSIS: HIGH RISK FOR INJURY *(CONTINUED)*

OUTCOME:

- The patient will be free from injury and able to function to the best of his or her abilities.

EVALUATION CRITERIA:

- There is no report or evidence of physical injury.
- There is no report or evidence of falls.

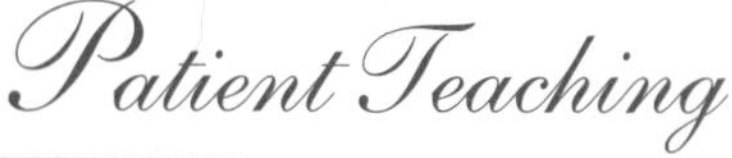

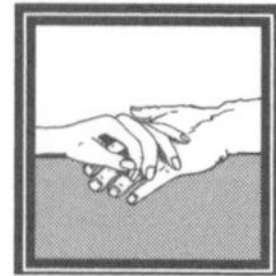

The prevention of falls should be the focus of your teaching interventions. It may not be possible to prevent every fall for every patient, but a significant reduction in the number and severity of falls can be achieved through an accurate assessment of a patient's risk factors and interventions designed to minimize them.

Emphasize that although it may seem that restraining the patient will eliminate the problem of falling, injuries are more likely to occur when the patient's mobility is restricted.

Environmental changes are a key element in fall prevention. Making some small changes can increase the patient's safety a great deal.

Explain to the patient or to family and other caregivers the importance of maintaining well-lighted, clutter-free passageways.

Eliminate such hazards as throw rugs, uneven flooring, slick surfaces, loose electrical cords, and small furniture items such as footstools.

Ensure that the patient's footwear fits well and is in good repair.

Stress the importance of moving deliberately and avoiding sudden attempts to stand or change position. Taking the time to sit on the edge of the bed before getting out of the bed may be all that's needed to decrease the incidence of postural hypotension and vertigo or syncope.

Instruct the patient in the proper use of assistive devices. Improper use may result in the patient's tripping over his or her own cane or walker.

Instruct family members to move carefully and deliberately around the patient at risk for falls. Encourage young children to allow the patient clear passage. Be alert to the presence of household pets because the patient can trip on them.

Encourage the patient to ask for help when necessary. Explain that you will try to anticipate his or her needs as much as possible, but that a little patience will pay off in reduced risk of injury.

If the patient does fall or has a near fall, attend to his or her immediate needs. Once the patient has recovered or has been treated, use the situation as an opportunity for developing interventions for "the next time." Encourage the patient to retain as much independence as possible, and stress the fact that one fall need not mean the end of all activity.

Documentation

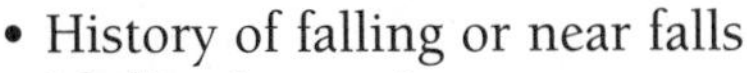

- History of falling or near falls
- Medication regimen
- Identification of a patient as at risk for falling
- Factors that may affect the patient's stability and increase the risk of falling
- Patient compliance with interventions

Nursing Research

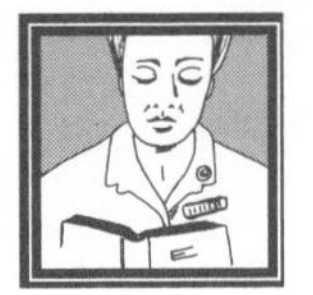

Studies show that an established fall prevention program that involves all members of staff—not just nursing staff—can significantly reduce the number of falls. This, in turn, reduces the threat of serious injury and death.

Brady, Rebecca, Frances R. Chester, Linda L. Pierce, Judith P. Salter, Sharon Schreck, and Roseanne Radziewicz. "Geriatric Falls: Prevention Strategies for the Staff." *Journal of Gerontological Nursing* 19 (September 1993): 26–32.

Chapter 6. Functional Decline and Immobility

Introduction

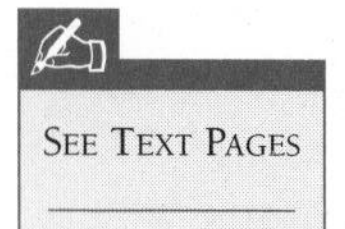

Although everyone experiences changes with aging, it is not a given that those changes must result in a decline in function. In fact, research has shown that an active lifestyle that includes physical exercise, social interaction, and emotionally satisfying relationships helps to prolong independence, foster good health, increase the ability to withstand and recover from illness, and improve the quality of life.

From the start, focus your patient interactions, interventions, and instruction on what the patient can do, not on what he or she cannot do. Concentrate on setting and achieving goals, not on following the path of least resistance toward maximum requirements for assistance.

Like so many other aspects of geriatric patient care, preventing functional decline is a balancing act. On the one hand, you want to emphasize ability, not disability, but on the other hand, you want to provide tools and techniques to make life easier for your patient.

You must also take measures when treating your patient in an acute situation to reduce the deleterious effects your interventions may have on other areas of the patient's functionality. For example, while a patient is immobilized for treatment of a broken hip, he or she may suffer from social withdrawal because the ability to visit friends may be limited.

Functional Decline Indicators

The following skills commonly are included in an evaluation of functional status:

- Bathing
- Dressing
- Grooming
- Eating
- Mobility
- Toileting

An evaluation of these activities of daily living (ADLs) may be expanded to include skills in communication, financial management, home care and maintenance, and other indicators of an independent life.

Research shows that for accurate assessment and effective intervention, these activities need to be considered in finer detail *and* as part of a bigger picture.

If assessment is limited to answering a question such as "Can this patient groom himself or herself adequately?" quite often the patient is rated poorly. Interventions may then be applied that support the assessment that the patient requires total assistance with grooming.

However, the patient might be able to complete some of the smaller tasks involved in grooming without aid and some with verbal prompting and be unable to manage only a few tasks. An assessment designed to identify these variations yields a clearer picture of the patient's actual abilities. This, in turn, allows the nursing staff to use specific interventions to help with certain areas, set clearly identifiable goals for improvement, and more easily measure progress toward those goals.

This finer-detail assessment has two parts: breakdown of a general task, such as grooming or toileting, into its components and use of a scale that more closely measures the level of assistance.

In the opposite direction, ADLs must be considered part of a bigger picture. If a patient cannot satisfactorily manage tasks involved in bathing, he or she might neglect grooming tasks, believing that "it's not worth brushing dirty hair."

Success in completing one ADL should be considered a stepping stone to success in completing other ADLs. Interventions should reinforce the patient's abilities and encourage the patient to extend himself or herself to succeed in other areas.

Benefits of Mobility

Mobility can be considered the underpinning of an independent existence. Positive effects that result from maintaining mobility include the following:

- Higher quality of life
- Enhanced self-image
- Lessened anxiety
- Reduced fatigue
- Greater stamina
- Increased resistance to disease
- Improved ability to recover from injury or illness

Helping your patient maintain his or her mobility may require some rethinking about mobility exercises. Although benefit can be achieved through physical therapy sessions, a better approach is to incorporate mobility practice and goals into all daily activities.

Every opportunity should be taken to reinforce the patient's ability to ambulate. Again, if the task is broken down into its components, patients and caregivers can focus on capabilities, goals, and improvements. This collaboration includes contributions from the following groups:

- Physical therapy staff, who evaluate the patient's capabilities, set goals for the patient, train other staff members in effective walking techniques, and periodically re-evaluate the patient
- Nursing staff, who encourage the patient to maintain mobility; develop ways to incorporate ambulation into the patient's daily care; share evaluation information, successes, and techniques with other staff members; and reinforce the importance of maintaining mobility with the patient, his or her caregivers, and other staff members
- Nonprofessional staff, who support the goals set by the nursing and physical therapy staff and work these goals into their interactions with the patient
- Family and other caregivers, who encourage the patient in his or her efforts and provide support for the patient in all efforts to maintain independence

NURSING DIAGNOSIS: HIGH RISK FOR ACTIVITY INTOLERANCE

RELATED TO:

- *Decreased physical fitness*

Nursing Interventions	Rationales
• Assess the patient's abilities to participate in exercise or walking programs.	• To determine the level of exertion the patient can expend
• Encourage the patient to participate in physical activities to the best of his or her abilities.	• To increase mobility
• Monitor the patient's vital signs before and after specific activities on a regular basis, such as weekly.	• To monitor activity intolerance and note improvements over baseline measurements
• Adjust the patient's daily routine to include mobility exercises. For example, encourage patients to walk to the dining room or to other areas independently.	• To reinforce the importance of maintaining mobility
• Plan walking or other exercise sessions to coincide with times of optimum functioning for the patient.	• To gain the maximum benefit from the exercise
• Help the patient to set realistic goals for physical fitness, and support the patient's efforts to reach those goals.	• To encourage patient participation in the care regimen

COLLABORATIVE MANAGEMENT

Interventions	Rationales
• Consult with physical therapy staff concerning patient abilities, goals, exercise levels, and progress.	• To develop an individualized program of fitness for the patient

NURSING DIAGNOSIS: HIGH RISK FOR ACTIVITY INTOLERANCE (CONTINUED)

COLLABORATIVE MANAGEMENT *(CONTINUED)*

Interventions *(continued)*	Rationales *(continued)*
• Consult with physical or occupational therapy staff about devices to support the patient's mobility, such as a cane.	• To provide options for the patient to consider
• Encourage the patient's family and other caregivers to support the patient's efforts to remain fit and to make opportunities to involve the patient in physical activities.	• To increase the likelihood that the patient will follow the fitness plan
• Administer medications, as ordered: analgesics.	• To reduce pain, which may prevent the patient from participating in fitness programs
• Provide information about the benefits of patient mobility to other staff members, and encourage their participation in patient fitness efforts.	• To involve all staff members in the program and increase the likelihood that the patient will receive maximum benefit

OUTCOME:	EVALUATION CRITERIA:
• The patient will maintain as much independent ambulation as possible.	• The patient meets or exceeds goals for ambulation as set by the physical therapy staff. • The patient can complete ADLs to the best of his or her ability.

NURSING DIAGNOSIS: SELF-CARE DEFICIT (DRESSING, GROOMING)

RELATED TO:

- *Decreased physical functioning*

Nursing Interventions	Rationales
• Assess the patient's abilities in completing dressing and grooming tasks.	• To determine where to focus your interventions
• Provide the minimum level of assistance required to help the patient complete the task. Assistance may involve the following: – Verbal cues, such as "It's time to put your shoes on" – Physical cues, such as touching the patient's arm to remind him or her of the task at hand – Modeling the task, hand over hand, to reinforce the behavior – Completing the task entirely	• To assure that the patient is adequately dressed and groomed, while encouraging him or her to complete as much of the task as possible
• Encourage the patient to choose the clothes he or she will wear. Reinforce the choices with positive comments about the patient's appearance.	• To increase the patient's self-esteem and reinforce his or her independence
• Teach ways to dress that take into account the patient's physical limitations. For example, instruct a patient to insert the less mobile limb into the garment first.	• To improve the chances for success in dressing
• Encourage the patient or caregiver to introduce the use of Velcro closures on clothing or to modify the patient's clothing in other ways that make it easier for the patient to manage.	• To compensate for diminshed dexterity and flexibility that can cause problems when dressing

NURSING DIAGNOSIS: SELF-CARE DEFICIT (DRESSING, GROOMING) (CONTINUED)

COLLABORATIVE MANAGEMENT

Interventions	Rationales
• Consult with physical and occupational therapy staff about devices the patient can use to make dressing and grooming easier.	• To provide additional options for the patient
• Provide suggestions to the patient, family, or other caregivers for modifying garments.	• To decrease the difficulty involved in dressing and grooming tasks

OUTCOME:	EVALUATION CRITERIA:
• The patient will complete activities involved in grooming and dressing.	• The patient is well groomed and neatly dressed. • The patient reports success with his or her ability to complete dressing and grooming tasks.

Patient Teaching

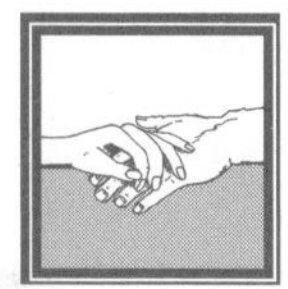

Emphasize that the patient is expected to complete tasks involved in ADLs to the best of his or her ability. This emphasis must be communicated to the patient, the nursing and other staff members, and the patient's family and other caregivers to avoid presentation of conflicting information to the patient.

Remind the staff and the patient's family and caregivers of the following benefits of maintaining patient independence:
- Increased quality of life for the patient
- Reduced workload for caregivers
- Increased time for nursing staff to spend on other patient care activities

Present information about devices, tools, and techniques for coping with changes in the patient's physical abilities. Such things include the following:
- Clothing altered or designed:
  - To permit room for and access to assistive devices

  - To allow easy manipulation
  - To accommodate physical changes, such as a thicker waist or spine curvature
  - To eliminate irritation from rough edges, seams, or texture
- Devices to improve reach and grasp, such as:
  - Extension pincers
  - Rods with a hook or loop on one end, such as the buttonhook illustrated below
  - Long-handled shoehorns, bath brushes, combs, or back scratchers
- Adaptations of commonly used items, such as:
  - Large-button telephones and television remote controls
  - Double-handled mugs
  - Easy-to-open medication containers
  - Large-print materials

ADAPTIVE DEVICES

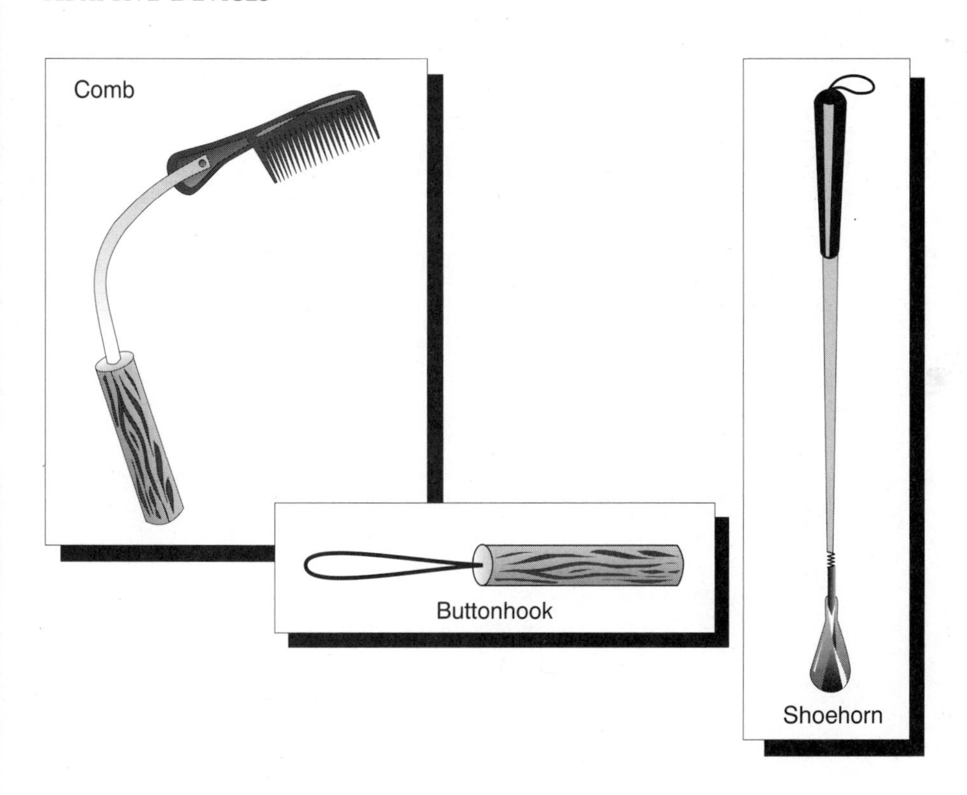

Documentation

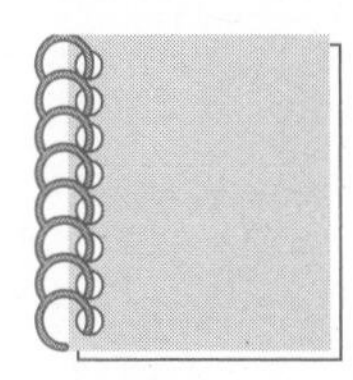

- Patient's functional status in completing ADLs
- Goals set by physical therapist for patient
- Patient's progress toward goals

Nursing Research

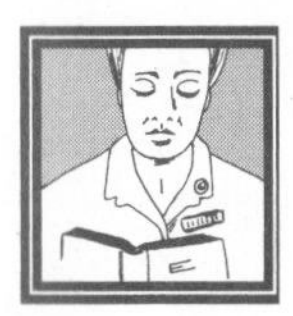

The application of uniform nursing interventions for all patients may not provide the best care for your patients. Studies show that many patients can do more for themselves when nursing staff provides assistance in response to specific needs instead of providing complete assistance. In other words, when caregivers resist the urge to "do it myself because it's quicker," the patient realizes greater benefit.

Osborn, C. L., and M. J. Marshall. "Self-Feeding Performance in Nursing Home Residents." *Journal of Geriatric Nursing* 19, no. 3 (1993): 7–14.

Chapter 7. Incontinence

Introduction

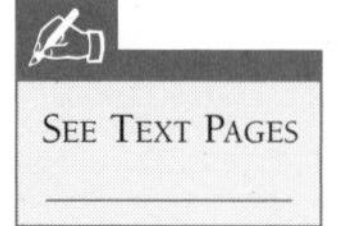

Urinary incontinence is prevalent among elderly people, with estimates placing its occurrence at more than 50% of nursing home residents and 30% of home-dwelling elders. However, it should not be considered a natural result of aging or impervious to treatment.

Many options are available to patients who suffer from this problem. Often the first step is uncovering the problem. Many people are unwilling to report the problem because of embarrassment or because they are afraid that it may be the beginning of unavoidable decline.

Once incontinence is reported or detected, a physical assessment must be completed to determine whether or not a medical condition is causing the problem. Many factors can cause or contribute to incontinence. They include medications, urinary tract infection, bowel impaction, and inadequate diet, especially fluid and fiber intake.

CAUSES OF INCONTINENCE

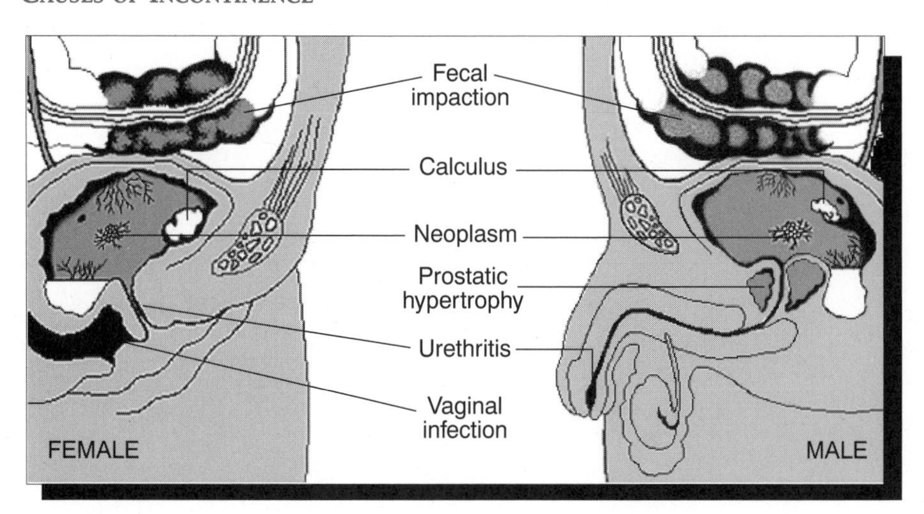

Types of Incontinence

Interventions for incontinence may vary, depending on the type. Many patients experience mixed incontinence—that is, a combination of types.

Stress incontinence occurs during incidents of strain on the supporting musculature, such as when a person coughs, sneezes, laughs, hiccups, or lifts a heavy object.

Urge incontinence occurs when the impulse to void is strong and sudden and the person does not have enough time to reach a toilet before voiding.

Reflex incontinence is similar to urge incontinence in that a person cannot reach toileting facilities in time to prevent an accident. This occurs, however, because the person does not experience the normal sensory signals that indicate a need to void.

Overflow incontinence occurs when there is a mechanical deficiency in the operation of the bladder or urethra which prevents adequate emptying of the bladder, such as enlarged prostrate, cerebrovascular accident, and fecal impaction. Unlike stress, urge, and reflex incontinence, overflow incontinence is not a sudden release of urine but is characterized by a constant leakage or dribbling of urine. Because of the potential for kidney damage, this condition should be evaluated immediately.

Functional incontinence is not caused by a deficiency in urinary function. Instead, it occurs when the patient is unable to complete the tasks associated with toileting because of dementia, functional or sensory impairments, immobility, or environmental constraints.

Interventions and treatment fall into the following basic categories:

- Behavioral strategies
- Pharmacologic therapies
- Surgical measures
- Use of containment devices

Whatever measures are taken, keep in mind the goals of restoring patient control, enhancing patient self-esteem, and respecting the patient's need for dignity, privacy, and choice.

Behavioral Strategies

Many patients resolve incontinence problems through behavior modification alone. The following are common behavioral strategies:

- Pelvic muscle exercises (Kegel exercises)
- Bladder retraining
- Dietary modification
- Habit training
- Relaxation technique training
- Biofeedback

Pharmacologic Strategies

Strategies that involve medication require an assessment of both the patient's need for drugs to manage the incontinence problem and the possibility that the drugs the patient is already taking for other ailments are causing the incontinence problem.

Drugs commonly used to treat incontinence include the following:

- Estrogen, which restores elasticity and moisture to the urethra, improving its function
- Antispasmodics, which help to relax the bladder, decrease urge sensations, and increase bladder capacity
- Sympathomimetics, which increase urethral closure strength
- Anticholinergics, which block contraction of the bladder

Drugs that may cause incontinence problems include the following:

- Diuretics, which cause the kidneys to produce larger quantities of urine
- Sedatives, which allow the patient to sleep so deeply that voiding urges are not felt or cause daytime drowsiness, which interferes with the patient's reaching the toilet in sufficient time
- Anticholinergics, which can lead to constipation and fecal impaction

Surgical Strategies

Although a nurse cannot surgically correct a patient's incontinence problem, interventions can be focused on educating the patient, family, and caregivers about surgical options; preparing the patient for surgery; and managing postoperative procedures.

Containment Devices

Devices to contain urine can be used while other methods are implemented to correct the problem or if the problem cannot be completely resolved. The choice of the device is governed by several factors, including patient characteristics such as size, functional status, and patterns of incontinence; availability and financial considerations; and caregiver or patient ability to manage the device.

Containment devices fall into the following general categories:
- Disposable protective devices that are designed to protect the patient's clothing and furniture from urine
- External collection devices, such as condom catheters
- Indwelling catheters

NURSING DIAGNOSIS: FUNCTIONAL INCONTINENCE

RELATED TO:
- *Environmental factors*

Nursing Interventions	Rationales
• Maintain the patient's micturition record or teach the patient to record the information.	• To determine actual voiding patterns
• Provide easy access to toileting facilities. Remove obstacles such as furniture and care equipment.	• To reduce access time to toileting facilities
• Ensure that the patient's bathroom is large enough to maneuver canes, walkers, or wheelchairs, if appropriate.	• To remove additional obstacles to toileting
• Provide adequate lighting with easily accessible switches or motion-sensitive lights.	• To reduce problems associated with poor illumination

Nursing Interventions *(continued)*	Rationales *(continued)*
• Encourage the patient to void at regular intervals, usually every 2 hours.	• To encourage development of a voiding schedule
• Encourage the patient to wear clothing that is easy to manipulate. Velcro closures, elastic waists, lengthened fly openings, and side-opening waistbands are some modifications that can be made to clothing to improve access.	• To reduce additional obstacles to toileting
• Examine the chairs or sofas on which the patient customarily sits. Ensure that the patient can easily rise from the seat. Floor-to-knee height should be appropriate for the patient, and the seat itself should be sturdy and tip-resistant.	• To avoid injury and delay as the patient attempts to rise

COLLABORATIVE MANAGEMENT

Interventions	Rationales
• Consult with the health care provider about any underlying diseases that might be causing incontinence.	• To identify other reasons for the patient's incontinence
• Consult with the pharmacist to determine if any medications are likely to be causing incontinence.	• To identify other reasons for the patient's incontinence

OUTCOME:	EVALUATION CRITERIA:
• The patient will void the appropriate amount of urine using toileting facilities and reduce or eliminate accidents.	• The patient reports satisfaction with adaptation to continence requirements. • The patient remains dry and comfortable. • The patient voids an adequate amount each day.

NURSING DIAGNOSIS: FUNCTIONAL INCONTINENCE

RELATED TO:

- *Cognitive impairment*

Nursing Interventions	Rationales
• Maintain the patient's micturition record.	• To determine actual voiding patterns
• Provide easy access to toileting facilities. Remove obstacles such as furniture and care equipment.	• To reduce access time to toileting facilities
• Identify toileting facilities clearly. Leave doors open and lights on.	• To encourage patients to use toileting facilities
• Remove potentially confusing objects from the bathroom, such as wastebaskets placed near toilets or urinals or mirrors, which may confuse the patient who may think someone is already using the facilities or is watching him or her.	• To reduce problems associated with the patient's confusion
• Encourage the patient to void at regular intervals.	• To encourage development of a voiding schedule
• When assisting a patient, provide clear, concise instructions in a calm, unhurried manner.	• To reduce patient confusion
• Encourage the patient to wear clothing that is easy to manipulate. Velcro closures, elastic waists, lengthened fly openings, and side-opening waistbands are some modifications that can be made to clothing to improve access.	• To reduce additional obstacles to toileting

COLLABORATIVE MANAGEMENT

Interventions	Rationales
• Consult with the health care provider about any underlying diseases that might be causing incontinence.	• To identify other reasons for the patient's incontinence
• Consult with pharmacist to determine if any medications are likely to cause incontinence.	• To identify other reasons for the patient's incontinence

OUTCOME:	EVALUATION CRITERIA:
• The patient will void the appropriate amount of urine using toileting facilities and reduce or eliminate accidents.	• The patient remains dry and comfortable. • The patient's skin shows no signs of irritation or breakdown. • The patient voids an adequate amount each day.

NURSING DIAGNOSIS: REFLEX INCONTINENCE

RELATED TO:

- *Absence of normal bladder sensation*

Nursing Interventions	Rationales
• Maintain the patient's micturition record.	• To determine actual voiding patterns
• Instruct the patient to perform pelvic muscle exercises on a regular schedule. An optimum schedule is a set of 10 to 25 repetitions done every other day.	• To improve muscle tone and control
• Encourage the patient to drink a sufficient amount of fluid (1,500 to 2,000 mL daily), unless contraindicated by other conditions, such as congestive heart failure.	• To reduce highly concentrated urine and stimulate the bladder-emptying response
• Encourage the patient to void on a regular schedule.	• To reduce accidents

NURSING DIAGNOSIS: REFLEX INCONTINENCE *(CONTINUED)*

Nursing Interventions *(continued)*	Rationales *(continued)*
• Instruct the patient in the use of self-catheterization equipment, if required.	• To completely empty the bladder

NURSE ALERT:
An indwelling catheter should be used only if the patient's incontinence interferes with the healing of pressure ulcers or during the immediate postoperative period. If a catheter must be used, clean, intermittent catheterization is the preferred method.

Nursing Interventions	Rationales
• If the patient is catheterized, be sure to maintain the urine flow into a drainage container. Inspect the tubing for bends or kinks, and empty the collection container regularly.	• To avoid bacterial contamination
• Provide catheter care, as defined by your institution's protocol.	• To reduce the risk of bacterial contamination
• Clean the patient immediately after an episode of fecal incontinence.	• To avoid bacterial contamination
• Follow infection control protocol and universal precautions when handling elements of the catheter system.	• To reduce the risk of infection
• Clean and dry the perineal area completely. Limit the number of catheter changes, and use the smallest effective catheter size.	• To avoid undue irritation

COLLABORATIVE MANAGEMENT

Interventions	Rationales
• Consult with the health care provider to schedule the patient for evaluation for a urinary tract infection.	• To identify and resolve any underlying urinary tract infection, of which incontinence is often a symptom

OUTCOME:

- The patient will void the appropriate amount of urine using toileting facilities and reduce or eliminate accidents.

EVALUATION CRITERIA:

- The patient or caregiver reports satisfaction with adaptation to continence requirements.
- The patient remains dry and comfortable.
- The patient voids an adequate amount each day.

NURSING DIAGNOSIS: STRESS INCONTINENCE

RELATED TO:

- *Weakened puboccygus muscles or dysfunctional urethral sphincter*

Nursing Interventions	Rationales
• Maintain the patient's micturition record.	• To determine actual voiding patterns
• Assess the patient for stress incontinence problems, including identification of physical activities that cause incontinence episodes.	• To determine where to focus your interventions
• Instruct the patient to perform pelvic muscle exercises on a regular schedule. An optimum schedule is a set of 10 to 25 repetitions done every other day.	• To improve muscle tone and control
• Encourage the patient to drink a sufficient amount of fluid (1,500 to 2,000 mL daily).	• To reduce highly concentrated urine and stimulate the bladder-emptying response

NURSING DIAGNOSIS: STRESS INCONTINENCE *(continued)*

Nursing Interventions *(continued)*	Rationales *(continued)*
• Encourage the patient to void on a regular schedule.	• To reduce accidents
• Instruct the patient in the use of containment or other protective devices, if required.	• To ensure adequate protection

COLLABORATIVE MANAGEMENT

Interventions	Rationales
• Consult with the health care provider about medical or surgical options for correcting incontinence.	• To provide additional options for the patient
• Consult with the health care provider to schedule the patient for evaluation for a urinary tract infection.	• To identify and resolve problems that may be causing incontinence

OUTCOME:

- The patient will void the appropriate amount of urine using toileting facilities and reduce or eliminate accidents.

EVALUATION CRITERIA:

- The patient or caregiver reports satisfaction with adaptation to continence requirements.
- The patient remains dry and comfortable.
- The patient voids an adequate amount each day.

NURSING DIAGNOSIS: URGE INCONTINENCE

RELATED TO:

- *Hyperactivity of the bladder*

Nursing Interventions	Rationales
• Maintain the patient's micturition record.	• To determine actual voiding patterns
• Instruct the patient to perform pelvic muscle exercises on a regular schedule and when the urge to void occurs. An optimum schedule is a set of 10 to 25 repetitions done every other day.	• To improve muscle tone and control and reduce the urge reflex
• Encourage the patient to drink a sufficient amount of fluid (1,500 to 2,000 mL daily). If necessary, limit intake during the 2 hours before bedtime.	• To reduce highly concentrated urine, stimulate the bladder-emptying response, and reduce nocturia
• Encourage the patient not to rush to the bathroom at the first urge impulse. Encourage the patient to control the urge through relaxation and pelvic muscle exercises and to move to the bathroom after the urge has passed.	• To use bladder relaxation techniques and reduce the occurrence of accidents on the way to the bathroom
• Encourage the patient to void on a regular schedule.	• To reduce accidents
• Instruct the patient in the use of relaxation exercises.	• To reduce the urge reflex

COLLABORATIVE MANAGEMENT

Interventions	Rationales
• Consult with the health care provider about medical and surgical options for correcting incontinence.	• To provide additional options for the patient

NURSING DIAGNOSIS: URGE INCONTINENCE *(CONTINUED)*

COLLABORATIVE MANAGEMENT *(CONTINUED)*

Interventions *(continued)*	Rationales *(continued)*
• Consult with the health care provider to schedule the patient for evaluation for a urinary tract infection.	• To identify and resolve problems that may be causing incontinence

OUTCOME:

- The patient will void the appropriate amount of urine using toileting facilities and reduce or eliminate accidents.

EVALUATION CRITERIA:

- The patient or caregiver reports satisfaction with adaptation to continence requirements.
- The patient remains dry and comfortable.
- The patient voids an adequate amount each day.

Patient Teaching

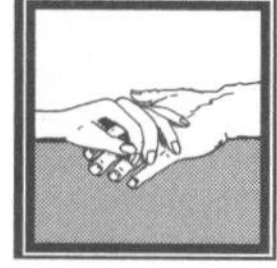

Emphasize to all geriatric patients, regardless of the type of incontinence they suffer or the cause of their problem, that incontinence is not a requirement of aging, that it responds well to treatment and intervention, and that it can be controlled to avoid a decrease in the quality of life.

Explain the relation between fluid and dietary intake and incontinence. Although it may seem logical to reduce intake to avoid accidents, this may cause problems by increasing the risk of constipation and the concentration of urine, thereby increasing irritation. Caffeine and artificial sweeteners can increase the frequency and urge for urination. Limiting intake before bedtime may reduce episodes of nocturia. Such a limitation is acceptable, provided sufficient fluids are consumed during daytime hours.

Pelvic muscle exercises can help to improve muscle tone and retention ability. Instruct the patient to perform these exercises on a regular basis. The following are simplified instructions for these exercises.

- Identify the muscles involved by voluntarily stopping a stream of urine.
- Once the muscle is located (but not while attempting to void), tighten it and hold it for a count of 10. If 10 seconds is too long, start with a 5-second hold. Relax the muscle for the same count.
- Repeat the exercises in a series of 10 at least three times a day.
- Don't use leg or stomach muscles to increase the muscle contraction. Remember to breathe regularly during the exercises.

Bladder retraining helps to increase the amount of time between voiding by using relaxation techniques. The following are simplified instructions for bladder retraining.

- If you experience an urge to void and fewer than 2½ hours have passed since you last voided, relax, breathe deeply, and complete at least one repetition of the pelvic muscle exercise to reduce the urge to void. Sit down during this period, if possible.
- Concentrate on taking slow, deep breaths and relaxing to eliminate the urge.
- Wait 5 minutes after the urge has passed or diminished and go to the bathroom. Go, even if you feel that you do not have to go. This will prevent the next urge from being too strong to avoid an accident.
- If you cannot wait 5 minutes and have an accident, shorten the waiting period to 3 minutes.
- Gradually increase the waiting time from 3 to 5 minutes and then to 10 minutes.

Habit training is useful with patients who are cognitively impaired or who suffer from reflex incontinence. This training is not aimed at altering bladder function. Rather, it is to develop a voiding habit that should eliminate accidents by having the patient void frequently. Simplified instructions for habit training are as follows.

- Go to the bathroom to pass urine every 2 hours whether you feel the urge or not. (A caregiver who is responsible for a cognitively impaired patient should set a 2-hour schedule for bathroom trips. This also provides an opportunity for mobility exercises.)
- If the urge to void occurs before the 2 hours pass, go then, but keep to your schedule.
- Complete your voiding diary for every attempt. This helps to determine your actual patterns of need and frequency.

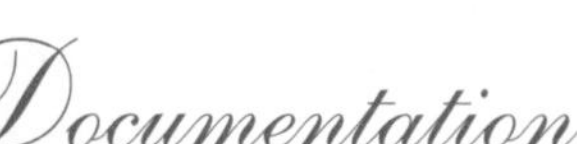

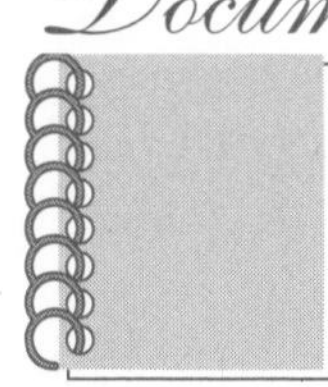

- Fluid intake and output
- Voiding patterns: frequency, schedule (after meals, on rising, and so forth)
- Bowel function
- Underlying conditions that affect continence
- Cognitive status
- Occurrence of accidents, including amount and possible causes

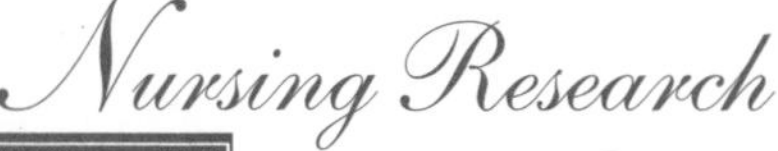

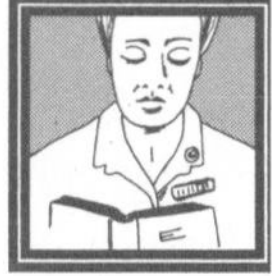

Research has shown that patients with cognitive impairment require additional time and attention to complete tasks related to toileting. Success in completing tasks related to one activity of daily living (ADL) encourages success in completing tasks related to other ADLs. Therefore, interventions aimed at increasing overall functionality may decrease incontinence episodes.

Morris, A., G. Browne, and A. Saltmarche. "Urinary Incontinence: Correlates Among Cognitively Impaired Elderly Veterans." *Journal of Gerontological Nursing* 18, no. 10 (1992): 33–42.

Chapter 8. Confusion

Introduction

SEE TEXT PAGES ______

Confusion is a general term used to describe the primary mental disorders that can afflict a geriatric patient. These disorders are more accurately termed delirium and dementia.

Delirium

Delirium, or acute confusional state, is a transient clinical state in which the patient may experience the following symptoms:

- Attention span disturbances, usually inattention
- Altered levels of consciousness, including drowsiness and lethargy as well as overalertness and insomnia
- Perceptual disturbances, such as hallucinations, nightmares, and illusions
- Reversal of diurnal cycle with periods of wakefulness during the night and sleep during the day
- Incoherent speech, thinking, and activity
- Emotional lability, including episodes of rage, fear, and extreme anxiety

The patient suffering from delirium often displays these symptoms suddenly. After this sudden onset, the symptoms fluctuate, making it difficult for caregivers to anticipate and cope with the effects of the disorder. Most deliriums are reversible, provided the condition is recognized and treated quickly. Conditions that may cause delirium include electrolyte imbalance, adverse drug reactions, dehydration, and infection.

Dementia

Dementia is seldom reversible. More than 70 conditions can cause dementia. Some specific dementias include Alzheimer's disease, Parkinson's disease, and AIDS-related dementia. The patient suffering from dementia may display the following symptoms:

- Memory impairment, usually for recent events, although as the disease progresses, long-term memories are lost as well

- Personality disorders, including behaviors that are inconsistent with the patient's history, a lack of concern for others, and inappropriate social behaviors
- Disturbances in cognitive functions, such as abstract reasoning, judgment, and insight
- Problems in communicating as language skills deteriorate
- Perception difficulties, including misinterpretations of environmental elements such as pictures or television images, inadequate depth perception, and misunderstanding of speech

The cause of dementia is varied, and it is complicated by the insidious nature of the symptoms. Caregivers may not recognize the gradual decline in the patient's abilities.

Superimposition of Delirium and Dementia

Delirium and dementia can be superimposed on each other, each exacerbating the symptoms of the other, making diagnosis difficult and posing great risk to the patient.

For example, a patient may exhibit what appear to be worsening symptoms of dementia when in reality, a change in medication or an illness has caused treatable and reversible delirium.

Dementia and delirium may appear similar in some ways. One difference is that the patient with dementia is usually awake and alert. The ongoing nature of dementia can mask the onset of life-threatening delirium, one of the reasons delirium is consistently underreported. Although delirium itself seldom causes death, the underlying illness or condition often escapes notice, so that delirium has to be considered a major cause of morbidity in geriatric patients.

The condition causing the delirium may also damage the patient's neuropsychological functioning to such a degree that even after the delirium is resolved, the patient still suffers from irreversible dementia.

Depression may also come into play in the patient suffering dementia. Symptoms of depression may appear to be signs of irreversible dementia. Depression is not limited to patients without dementia.

Safety Issues

For the health care professional treating patients suffering from delirium or dementia, the primary focus should be on ensuring patient safety with as little compromise to the patient's autonomy as possible.

Once the patient's safety is assured, interventions should center on maintaining as much functionality as possible for the patient with dementia and solving the underlying cause of the disorder for the patient suffering from delirium. This underlying cause can be an illness, a reaction to medication, or symptoms of depression, for example.

Measures to ensure safety must be designed to address the needs of the following people:

- The patient, who may view the measures as unwanted control and loss of autonomy and freedom
- The caregivers, who may view the measures as an additional burden and alteration in lifestyle
- The health care professionals, if the patient is in a hospital or nursing home environment, who may view the measures as difficult to apply to a variable patient population

The best care plan requires the adaptation of nursing and caregiver interventions to each patient, keeping in mind the goal of safety with as little cost to patient autonomy as possible.

Use and Abuse of Restraint

The use of patient restraint is central to the issue of safety versus autonomy. Restraint, whether physical or chemical, should be considered an extreme measure, to be applied in unusual circumstances.

Using restraints has an adverse effect on many patients, especially those suffering from delirium or dementia, who do not have the powers of reasoning to understand why they have been restrained.

In the struggle to free himself or herself, the patient may be injured or may injure others. The experience of being restrained may also decrease patient cooperation and increase patient anxiety.

The need for patient restraint can be reduced by the following means:

- Adapting the patient's physical environment to allow for safe wandering
- Decreasing the risks inherent in increased patient activity
- Providing proper postural support so that the patient can sit, rise, and transfer comfortably with minimal aid
- Addressing disruptive behaviors with an eye toward prevention
- Promoting patient functioning and focusing on what the patient can do, not on what he or she cannot do

Reorientation and Validation

The range of behavior in patients suffering from delirium or dementia is quite wide. Some may experience a slight disturbance in functioning, whereas others cannot function at all.

As you begin to tailor your care plan to meet the needs of an individual patient, you will need to determine your approach to the patient's perception of reality.

Reorientation

You may choose to *reorient* the patient to the current time, place, and circumstance. This usually is appropriate for patients who are in the early stages of dementia or who are recovering from the effects of delirium.

Reorientation may take the form of conversational cues, such as "Today is Friday, the day your sister comes to visit." In institutional settings, patients may be reminded of the day, date, time, season, or other general facts through the use of posters or signs.

Your efforts toward reorientation need not be obtrusive. In fact, repeated recitations of the date and time or repeated questioning of the patient about his or her name, for example, may increase patient anxiety and distress.

Validation

You may also choose to *validate* the patient's own perception of reality for several reasons.

- It decreases anxiety and agitation that may be caused by the patient's inability to understand your reorientation efforts.
- It may promote patient cooperation, allowing you to perform needed care or examinations.
- Reorientation may serve little purpose for the patient with severe perception difficulties. It would be wasted energy and effort on your part—energy you could expend in other caretaking activities.

Validation calls for you to enter the patient's reality to the extent that you can promote the patient's well-being, instruct the patient in performing self-care tasks, redirect the patient's unsafe or unwanted behavior, and acquire information from the patient about his or her condition.

For example, if a patient insists on completing the housework, ask her to help you with the laundry and set her to folding linens or towels.

If the patient refuses to eat because he can't pay the bill, tell him that it's part of the "package deal" or show him a paid receipt.

More than likely, your interventions will be a mix of these two techniques. Your choice will depend on your immediate goal in interacting with the patient and how that goal fits in with your long-term care plan.

Dealing with Disruptive Behavior

Despite efforts to maintain a safe environment for the patient, sometimes the patient may act in a violent, disturbed, or disruptive manner. Steps must be taken to prevent the patient from hurting himself or herself or others.

Preventing the disruptive behavior is by far the best method of managing the problem. As the health care professionals who are responsible for the patient get to know his or her habits, likes and dislikes, and anxiety triggers, the opportunities for heading off disruptive behavior increase. Caregivers at home can learn to take advantage of this knowledge as well.

Caregiver reaction may inadvertently reinforce the disruptive behavior. If the patient is feeling neglected or isolated and learns that a violent display of temper brings people running, it won't be long before that behavior becomes habitual. Although the patient should not be ignored or punished for disruptive behavior, the caregiver must learn to deal with the problem and concentrate positive attention and other rewards on acceptable behavior.

Consistency is a key element in dealing with a disruptive patient. Plans for managing the behavior must be clearly communicated to the staff, if the patient is in a hospital or nursing home, or to all caregivers in the patient's home.

Steps to Take

If the patient does display disruptive behavior, follow these steps to allow the patient to regroup and to prevent injury to the patient, other patients, the caregiver, or yourself.

- Face the patient directly, staying in his or her line of vision. Try not to approach the patient from behind.
- Maintain eye contact as long as this does not increase the patient's agitation.
- Speak calmly, clearly, and simply. State in short sentences exactly what you want the patient to do. Saying "Stop that!" to a patient who is yelling, pushing things to the floor, and looking around for his mother does not make clear to the patient what you want him to stop doing.
- Touch the patient gently on the arm or shoulder to redirect him or her away from the unsafe areas or the center of attention. Do not insist on maintaining contact if it frightens or distresses the patient.
- Try to identify the underlying cause for the distress and eliminate it.
- Avoid the impulse to rush the patient into compliance with your instructions.
- Limit the effect the patient's behavior has on others by asking people to leave, if possible, or by guiding the patient to a quiet area.
- Restraint of the patient, either physically or by using medication, is a last resort and should be used only when no other interventions are effective in preventing the patient from coming to or causing harm.

Once the disruptive episode is over, do not concentrate on it with the patient. Be sure to develop a plan to avoid future occurrences.

NURSING DIAGNOSIS: ALTERED FAMILY PROCESSES

RELATED TO:

- *Impaired cognitive abilities caused by dementia or delirium*

Nursing Interventions	Rationales
• Assess the patient's relationship with other members of her or his family.	• To determine the organization of the family and better focus your interventions
• Discuss with the patient and caregivers characteristics of the new roles the patient will take.	• To support the patient in the changing situation
• Encourage open communication between all family members.	• To prevent misunderstandings and additional stress
• Provide information about the patient's illness or condition to the family, using the appropriate language.	• To facilitate their decision making
• Recommend that the family take advantage of counseling and other support services, as applicable.	• To reduce stress on the patient and the family

COLLABORATIVE MANAGEMENT

Interventions	Rationale
• Consult with the psychiatric staff or social workers to discover other resources for the patient and family, such as support groups.	• To provide additional options for the family to consider

OUTCOME:	EVALUATION CRITERIA:
• The patient and his or her family will adjust to the new roles.	• The patient or caregiver reports satisfaction with the arrangements that have been made.
	• Obvious signs of disharmony, such as arguing, avoiding the patient, and noncompliance with arrangements, are absent.

NURSING DIAGNOSIS: IMPAIRED VERBAL COMMUNICATION

RELATED TO:

- *Brain damage caused by dementia or delirium*

Nursing Interventions	Rationales
• Address the patient in a clear, calm, low-pitched voice. Make sure the patient can see you clearly before you begin talking.	• To accommodate for hearing loss and compensate for brain damage that may be causing communication impairment
• Face the patient at his or her eye level. Crouch down to speak to the patient who is seated, for example.	• To avoid intimidation of the patient and to allow him or her to focus on your face
• Limit the amount of background noise, including television, public address systems, and the noise of routine activity.	• To reduce environmental press on the patient
• Wait patiently for the patient to form a response to your questions or comments.	• To avoid additional stress on the patient and allow enough time for the patient suffering from brain damage to process the information
• Limit your instructions to simple commands accompanied by gestures to assist the patient in understanding.	• To avoid confusing the patient and to provide cues that can help the patient compensate for his or her lost or impaired ability to process information
• Touch the patient in a nonthreatening way.	• To guide his or her actions and provide reassurance
• Use direct, yes-or-no questions.	• To reduce the risk of additional confusion
• Use terms that are familiar to the patient.	• To reduce the patient's effort to understand your instructions
• Avoid repeatedly correcting the patient or asking orientation questions.	• To limit patient frustration

Nursing Interventions *(continued)*	Rationales *(continued)*
• Identify behavioral cues that indicate the patient's boredom, stress, or frustration, and bring the conversation to a close before disruptive behavior occurs.	• To prevent the patient from engaging in inappropriate or unacceptable behavior

COLLABORATIVE MANAGEMENT

Interventions	Rationales
• Enlist the support of all staff members and family and other caregivers in a consistent approach to communicating with the patient.	• To reduce patient confusion over differing instructions or conversational styles
• Confer with hearing specialists to determine if the patient's hearing loss can be corrected.	• To remove physical barriers to effective communication

OUTCOME:	EVALUATION CRITERIA:
• Communication of instruction or information to the patient is adequate.	• Signs of frustration or agitation and catastrophic episodes are reduced or absent.

NURSING DIAGNOSIS: FLUID VOLUME DEFICIT

RELATED TO:

- *Illness or condition underlying the patient's delirium*

Nursing Interventions	Rationales
• Monitor the patient's fluid intake and output.	• To determine patterns of intake and output to more easily identify variations
• Weigh the patient regularly—daily or weekly—as his or her condition warrants.	• To detect fluid gains or losses

NURSING DIAGNOSIS: FLUID VOLUME DEFICIT *(CONTINUED)*

Nursing Interventions *(continued)*	Rationales *(continued)*
• Monitor the patient's blood pressure. Be sure to obtain readings when the patient is lying down, seated, and standing. If the patient cannot stand, be sure to take the other two readings.	• To provide an initial baseline and monitor any orthostatic changes
• Maintain the patency of I.V. lines and drainage tubes, if appropriate.	• To assure adequate fluid intake and output
• Obtain an accurate estimate of blood loss, if appropriate.	• To assure early detection of fluid volume deficit
• Assess for other signs of fluid volume deficit, such as altered mental status, increased anxiety, increased heart rate, poor skin turgor, dehydrated mucous membranes, and hypotension.	• To assure early detection of fluid volume deficit

COLLABORATIVE MANAGEMENT

Interventions	Rationales
• Assess laboratory values for complete blood count, creatinine and electrolyte levels, and baseline hematocrit and hemoglobin.	• To assure early detection of fluid volume deficit
• Assess the patient's central venous pressure (CVP) status.	• To assure early detection of fluid volume deficit
• Administer a blood or fluid transfusion, as ordered.	• To alleviate fluid volume deficit

OUTCOME:	EVALUATION CRITERIA:
• The patient will experience adequate fluid volume.	• Urine output is normal (>30 mL/hr.). • Serum electrolyte levels are within normal limits.

NURSING DIAGNOSIS: FLUID VOLUME DEFICIT (*CONTINUED*)

OUTCOME: (*CONTINUED*)	EVALUATION CRITERIA: (*CONTINUED*)
• The patient will experience adequate fluid volume. (*continued*)	• CVP is within normal limits.
	• Vital signs are stable.

NURSING DIAGNOSIS: FUNCTIONAL INCONTINENCE

RELATED TO:

- *Memory loss and cognitive and perceptual impairments experienced by patients suffering from dementia*

Nursing Interventions	Rationales
• Maintain the patient's micturition record.	• To determine actual voiding patterns
• Monitor fluid intake and output.	• To ensure adequate hydration
• Encourage the patient to void at regular intervals.	• To encourage development of a voiding schedule
• Identify the bathroom clearly, using signs with pictures or words.	• To establish landmarks for the patient
• Remove potentially confusing elements from the bathroom, such as wastebaskets near the toilet. Leave the toilet lid open.	• To give additional cues to the patient
• Encourage the patient to dress in clothing that is easy to manipulate.	• To decrease the patient's stress

COLLABORATIVE MANAGEMENT

Interventions	Rationales
• Obtain laboratory values, such as complete blood count and electrolyte levels.	• To rule out urinary tract infection as an underlying cause of incontinence

NURSING DIAGNOSIS: FUNCTIONAL INCONTINENCE *(CONTINUED)*

COLLABORATIVE MANAGEMENT *(CONTINUED)*

Interventions *(continued)*	Rationales *(continued)*
• Administer medications, as ordered: anticholinergics.	• To reduce the need for excessive voiding

NURSE ALERT:
Anticholinergics may cause constipation, fecal incontinence, urine retention, and dry mouth. Use these medications with care in an elderly patient.

Interventions *(continued)*	Rationales *(continued)*
• Consult with the therapy staff about methods the patient could use to manage his or her continence needs adequately.	• To provide additional options for the patient

OUTCOME:

- The patient will void the appropriate amount of urine within a reasonable pattern and will not experience adverse effects from using incontinence aids.

EVALUATION CRITERIA:

- Output is about 240 to 500 mL for each voiding episode.
- The patient's voiding pattern is about once every 2 to 4 hours and not more than once at night.
- The patient or caregiver reports satisfaction with adaptation to continence requirements.
- The patient remains dry and comfortable.
- The patient's fluid intake and output are relatively equal.
- The patient takes in adequate fluid to support tissue hydration.
- The patient voids an adequate amount each day.

NURSING DIAGNOSIS: HIGH RISK FOR INFECTION

RELATED TO:

- *Illness or condition underlying the patient's delirium*

Nursing Interventions	Rationales
• Assess the patient for pre-existing disposition to infection, especially the status of his or her immune system.	• To prevent onset or worsening of infection
• Monitor vital signs for changes that indicate infection, such as elevated temperature and rapid heart rate.	• To prevent onset or worsening of infection

NURSE ALERT:
In the elderly patient, symptoms of infection may not be clear-cut. For example, your patient might not exhibit a true temperature spike (101.5°F [38.6°C]) but still have an infection. Similarly, the patient who is taking beta blockers will not demonstrate tachycardia.

Nursing Interventions	Rationales
• Encourage the patient to drink fluids, maintain adequate nutrition, and rest frequently.	• To prevent onset or worsening of infection
• Teach the patient basic infection-control practices, such as hand washing and avoidance of other infected people.	• To minimize the risk of contracting infection
• Adhere to institutional protocol for infection control and sanitation.	• To reduce the risk of contracting infection

NURSING DIAGNOSIS: HIGH RISK FOR INFECTION *(CONTINUED)*

COLLABORATIVE MANAGEMENT

Interventions	Rationales
• Obtain a complete blood count with erythrocyte sedimentation rate.	• To evaluate potential infection

NURSE ALERT:
The atypical presentation of symptoms of infection in an elderly person may lead to inaccurate diagnosis of infection. For example, the patient's complete blood count may be only slightly elevated because some elderly people are unable to mount a significant leukocytosis, or the erythrocyte sedimentation rate may be elevated because of the presence of chronic inflammatory diseases.

Interventions	Rationales
• Administer medications, as ordered: antibiotics.	• To reduce or eliminate infection

NURSE ALERT:
Be careful to assess the patient for adverse reactions to drugs and food.

Interventions	Rationales
• Prepare the patient, if necessary, for surgery.	• To control infection

OUTCOME:	EVALUATION CRITERIA:
• The patient will show no signs of infection.	• Vital signs are normal.
	• Laboratory values are normal.

NURSING DIAGNOSIS: HIGH RISK FOR INJURY

RELATED TO:

- *Impaired judgment, loss of impulse control, and impaired cognitive abilities in patients suffering from delirium or dementia*

Nursing Interventions	Rationales
• Provide a safe environment in which the patient can wander or pace.	• To reduce the risk of injury or of the patient getting lost and disoriented
• Limit the use of restraints, either physical or chemical.	• To reduce the risk that the patient will suffer injury in trying to escape the physical restraint or in trying to function in a drugged state
• If the patient uses a hospital bed, lower the side rails and the bed itself, if possible.	• To reduce the risk of injury when the patient gets out of bed
• Use bed alarms that activate when the patient attempts to climb out of bed.	• To allow the staff to reach the patient in time to prevent a fall
• Reduce the amount of clutter or extraneous equipment in the patient's environment.	• To avoid confusing the patient or presenting too many obstacles for the patient to navigate safely
• Avoid changing the layout or location of the patient's room.	• To reduce patient confusion
• If the patient is cared for in the home environment, restrict access to tools or other dangerous implements; to hazardous areas such as garages, basements, and garden sheds; and to medications and cleaning supplies.	• To ensure patient safety
• If the patient is attempting to dislodge tubing or other iatrogenic devices, relocate them, if appropriate, to areas the patient cannot reach.	• To prevent injury from the forcible removal of iatrogenic devices

NURSING DIAGNOSIS: HIGH RISK FOR INJURY *(CONTINUED)*

COLLABORATIVE MANAGEMENT

Interventions	Rationales
• Consult with the physical or occupational therapy staff for activities to keep the patient occupied.	• To encourage patient participation in safe activities
• Consult with the physical or occupational therapy staff about devices that allow the patient movement but that limit access to iatrogenic devices.	• To reduce the risk of injury from the forcible removal of iatrogenic devices
• If the patient is cared for in a hospital or nursing home setting, post pictures of the patient at each station.	• To allow staff to recognize patients at risk for wandering behavior
• Provide some means of identifying the patient.	• To ensure that staff unfamiliar with the patient can help him or her return safely to living quarters
• Consult with the occupational therapy staff about alarms or other devices that can alert caregivers to patient activity.	• To more effectively monitor patient behavior

OUTCOME:

- The patient will be free from injury and able to function to the best of his or her abilities.

EVALUATION CRITERIA:

- There is no report or evidence of physical injury.
- Displays by the patient of frustrated or stressed behavior are decreased or absent.

NURSING DIAGNOSIS: ALTERED NUTRITION (LESS THAN BODY REQUIREMENTS)

RELATED TO:

- *Patient's agnosia, apraxia, or other perceptual deficiencies*

Nursing Interventions	Rationales
• Document the patient's weight, height, vital signs, and current nutritional status.	• To use as a baseline for evaluating patient status
• Monitor the patient's weight regularly—either daily or weekly—as the patient's condition warrants.	• To detect weight loss as quickly as possible
• Establish a consistent routine for mealtimes.	• To reduce patient confusion
• Identify techniques for increasing the likelihood that the patient will eat, such as preparing smaller, more frequent meals; preparing favorite foods often; limiting the number of choices confronting the patient at mealtime.	• To increase patient compliance with the nutritional plan
• Identify areas of potential harm to the patient, such as overheated food, overfilled cups or glasses, and sharp implements.	• To reduce the risk of injury

COLLABORATIVE MANAGEMENT

Interventions	Rationales
• Consult with the dietitian to develop a diet plan for the patient.	• To ensure adequate nu
• Monitor laboratory values, such as serum albumin and protein levels.	• To determine nutritional status and identify when supplements are needed
• Enlist the help of family members or other caregivers in making the dining experience pleasurable and comfortable for the patient.	• To promote patient compliance with the nutritional plan

NURSING DIAGNOSIS: ALTERED NUTRITION (LESS THAN BODY REQUIREMENTS) *(CONTINUED)*

COLLABORATIVE MANAGEMENT *(CONTINUED)*

Interventions *(continued)*	Rationales *(continued)*
• Administer nutritional supplements, as ordered.	• To ensure adequate nutrition

OUTCOME:	EVALUATION CRITERIA:
• The patient will maintain optimum weight and adequate nutritional status.	• Weekly weight gain is in accordance with set goals. • Nutritional status is at appropriate levels for the patient.

NURSING DIAGNOSIS: IMPAIRED PHYSICAL MOBILITY

RELATED TO:

- *Impairments in physical capability, perceptual disturbances, and decreased communication skills*

Nursing Interventions	Rationales
• Allow the patient freedom to wander and exercise safely.	• To avoid muscle atrophy
• Be alert to changes in the patient's physical activity that may signal fatigue, anxiety, adverse reaction to medication, [illegible]r pain and discomfort.	• To reduce the risk of injury
• [illegible]structing the patient to [illegible]n activity, model the [illegible]urself. For example, [illegible]nt the patient to sit [illegible], lead him or her to a [illegible]nd sit down in an adjacent chair.	• To reduce the effects of memory loss, apraxia, and agnosia
• Avoid restraining the patient.	• To reduce the risk of injury if the patient tries to escape the restraint

Nursing Interventions *(continued)*	Rationales *(continued)*
• Promote good posture and reduce muscle fatigue by using support pillows or cushions and comfortable chairs and beds.	• To reduce strain on muscles
• When working with a patient to complete exercises, allow the patient to complete as much of the exercise as possible.	• To achieve maximum benefit, even if the activity is minimal
• When a patient is hesitant to begin an activity, coach him or her with touch or verbal cues.	• To encourage the patient to do as much as possible for himself or herself
• If the patient can no longer walk, complete regular range-of-motion exercises.	• To reduce muscle atrophy

COLLABORATIVE MANAGEMENT

Interventions	Rationales
• Consult with the physical or occupational therapy staff for exercises to help the patient maintain muscle tone and mobility.	• To prevent decline into immobility
• Enlist the aid of the family and other caregivers in walking or exercising with the patient.	• To increase patient compliance with the physical therapy regimen

OUTCOME:	EVALUATION CRITERIA:
• The patient will maintain as much physical mobility as possible.	• The patient is able to ambulate with as little assistance as possible. • Evidence of physical complications of immobility, such as pressure ulcers, muscle atrophy, and injury, is decreased or absent.

NURSING DIAGNOSIS: SELF-CARE DEFICIT (TOTAL)

RELATED TO:

- *Impairments in physical capability, perceptual disturbances, and decreased communication skills*

Nursing Interventions	Rationales
• Concentrate on the patient's abilities to complete self-care tasks.	• To encourage the patient to do as much as possible for himself or herself
• Avoid completing the task yourself. Instead, assist or prompt the patient with touch or verbal cues.	• To decrease the patient's frustration and feeling of inadequacy
• Establish a routine for toileting activities, bathing, hair washing, and other self-care tasks.	• To decrease the patient's stress and anxiety over the self-care routines
• If a particular task is stressful for the patient, schedule it to take advantage of the patient's "good" time.	• To decrease stress on the patient and prevent catastrophic incidents
• Maintain a calm attitude toward the patient, respecting his or her privacy and dignity.	• To promote the patient's feeling of self-worth and confidence
• Compliment the patient on his or her grooming efforts.	• To increase patient compliance with the care routine

COLLABORATIVE MANAGEMENT

Interventions	Rationales
• Consult with the physical or occupational therapy staff about tools or devices that can make self-care tasks easier for the patient, such as long-handled brushes for cleaning the back, a stool or chair for use in the shower, and hand-held shower heads.	• To provide options for the patient
• Encourage the patient to dress in clothing that is easy to manipulate.	• To reduce the effort involved in self-care tasks

COLLABORATIVE MANAGEMENT *(CONTINUED)*

Interventions *(continued)*	Rationales *(continued)*
• Arrange for a hair dresser, dental hygienist, manicurist, or other technicians to help the patient maintain his or her appearance.	• To promote the patient's interest in self-care
• Consult with the health care provider about medications the patient is taking that might affect his or her appearance or hygiene requirements, such as hair loss from cancer treatments.	• To anticipate the need for special attention during self-care routines

OUTCOME:	EVALUATION CRITERIA:
• The patient will take as active a role as possible in his or her own care.	• The patient demonstrates ability to complete self-care tasks. • The patient displays a clean, neat, and well-groomed appearance.

NURSING DIAGNOSIS: SENSORY/PERCEPTUAL ALTERATIONS

RELATED TO:
- *Dementia or delirium*

Nursing Interventions	Rationales
• Assess the patient's sense of hearing, sight, touch, smell, taste, and motion.	• To determine the areas in which to focus your interventions
• If the patient has hearing problems, speak clearly in a low-pitched voice while directly facing the patient. Reduce background or ambient noise as much as possible. Accompany your speech with appropriate gestures.	• To increase the patient's ability to understand your speech

NURSING DIAGNOSIS: SENSORY/PERCEPTUAL ALTERATIONS (CONTINUED)

Nursing Interventions *(continued)*	Rationales *(continued)*
• If the patient has vision problems, provide adequate illumination, using nonglare lighting. Increase the contrast near dangerous areas, such as stairs and doorways. Evaluate the patient's environment for areas of shadow that might be misperceived by the patient.	• To increase the patient's ability to accurately see his or her environment
• If the patient has deficiencies in taste or smell, adapt the patient's meals to accommodate his or her altered senses. Provide familiar scents, such as cinnamon, bread, coffee, or tea.	• To promote patient interest in food and provide familiar olfactory sensations in an effort to reduce the risk of malnutrition
• If the patient suffers an impairment in the sense of touch or motion, adapt the patient's enviroment to take this into account. For example, install door handles that are levers, not knobs, and provide insulated cups to protect the patient from burns from hot beverages.	• To reduce the risk of injury

COLLABORATIVE MANAGEMENT

Interventions	Rationales
• Consult with the physical or occupational therapy staff about devices that can promote the patient's functioning despite impaired senses.	• To minimize the effect of sensory impairment on the patient's activities
• Schedule appointments with vision and hearing specialists.	• To determine if corrective devices are needed

COLLABORATIVE MANAGEMENT *(CONTINUED)*

Interventions *(continued)*	Rationales *(continued)*
• Collaborate with the physical or occupational therapist, the patient, and his or her caregivers, if appropriate, to evaluate the patient's environment for safety risks that a patient with sensory impairment might not perceive.	• To reduce the risk of injury
• Encourage the patient and family to take advantage of various support services for people with sensory impairment.	• To increase patient compliance with therapy designed to address sensory impairment
• Stress the importance of proper fit and the use of prosthetic sensory aids, such as hearing aids and eyeglasses.	• To increase the value of these devices to the patient

OUTCOME:	EVALUATION CRITERIA:
• The patient will experience minimal or no effect from sensory impairments.	• The patient sees clearly. • The patient hears clearly. • The patient's sense of smell or taste is accommodated through dietary or environmental changes. • The patient remains free from injury related to impairment of the sense of touch or motion. • The patient's environment is free from the hazards a patient suffering from impairment of one or more senses might not perceive.

NURSING DIAGNOSIS: SLEEP PATTERN DISTURBANCE

RELATED TO:

- *Disorientation caused by delirium or dementia*

Nursing Interventions	Rationales
• Assess the patient's current sleep patterns.	• To help the patient identify problem areas
• Encourage the patient to regulate sleeping patterns by rising at the same time every day and getting the same amount of rest each night.	• To develop good sleeping habits and strengthen circadian rhythms
• Limit caffeine intake, restrict exercise or activity to the morning or early afternoon, and prepare for sleep with routine tasks.	• To reduce external causes for disturbed sleep
• Discourage the use of alcohol as a sleeping aid.	• To reduce the risk of establishing a fragmented sleep pattern in which the patient falls to sleep quickly but often awakes and finds it difficult to return to sleep
• If sundowning is part of the sleep disturbance, encourage the patient to take a daytime nap. Fatigue may contribute to the sundown effect.	• To reduce overtiredness, which may result in insomnia
• Schedule nursing activities so that the patient can have an uninterrupted night's sleep.	• To encourage regular sleep patterns
• Provide a quiet, darkened room for sleep.	• To provide visual cues for the patient if he or she should awaken during the night
• Provide a nightlight in the patient's room.	• To orient the patient if he or she should awaken during the night

Nursing Interventions *(continued)*

- If the patient does wake up during the night, determine if he or she needs to use the bathroom or is hungry, thirsty, or in pain and address those needs.

Rationales *(continued)*

- To promote a return to restful sleep and decrease or alleviate anxiety caused by misperceptions of the environment

COLLABORATIVE MANAGEMENT

Interventions

- Consult with other health care providers for suggestions to regulate the patient's sleep patterns.
- Avoid medications, unless necessary.

Rationales

- To develop a plan for coping with altered sleep patterns
- To reduce the risk of injury if the patient attempts to get up unaided during the night and to reduce confusion and restlessness that may be an adverse effect of the medication

OUTCOME:

- The patient will experience restful, adequate sleep.

EVALUATION CRITERIA:

- The patient reports satisfaction with the amount of sleep and its quality.
- Signs of excessive fatigue or hyperactivity are decreased or absent.

NURSING DIAGNOSIS: IMPAIRED SOCIAL INTERACTION

RELATED TO:

- *Changes in personality caused by delirium or dementia*

Nursing Interventions	Rationales
• Encourage the patient to participate in as many activities as he or she is able to tolerate.	• To reduce loneliness and increase interaction

NURSE ALERT:
As the patient's dementia becomes more advanced, he or she may function best if interactions are limited to small groups of people.

Nursing Interventions	Rationales
• Engage the patient in normal conversation and interaction on a one-to-one basis.	• To encourage the patient to use his or her social skills
• Limit the amount of stimulus in the patient's environment.	• To avoid overstimulating the patient who is making tentative social contacts and to avoid catastrophic episodes
• Focus the patient on a specific activity that is appropriate for the patient's interests and functional capacity.	• To increase the patient's sense of self-worth and encourage involvement with others

COLLABORATIVE MANAGEMENT

Interventions	Rationales
• Consult with the occupational or physical therapists about activities in which the patient can participate with others.	• To encourage group involvement
• Encourage the patient's family or other caregivers to communicate with the patient frequently, either in person or over the phone.	• To decrease patient isolation

COLLABORATIVE MANAGEMENT *(CONTINUED)*

Interventions *(continued)*	Rationales *(continued)*
• Encourage staff members to include the patient in as many activities as possible within the patient's ability to tolerate such activity.	• To encourage patient participation in social interaction

OUTCOME:	EVALUATION CRITERIA:
• The patient will enjoy social interaction with family, friends, other patients, and staff to the best of his or her abilities.	• The patient enjoys interaction with others. • Frustrated or stressed behaviors or catastrophic episodes are reduced or absent.

NURSING DIAGNOSIS: ALTERED THOUGHT PROCESSES

RELATED TO:

- *Chronic dementia or the illness or condition underlying the patient's delirium*

Nursing Interventions	Rationales
• Assess the patient's perception of reality.	• To determine areas on which to focus your interventions
• Reduce the amount of environmental noise and activity.	• To allow the patient to focus on a few important elements of his or her environment
• If your care plans include reorientation, advise the patient of his or her status. Include such information as the following: – Location (hospital or nursing home, for example) – Reason the patient is there – Day, date, time, season, or other significant temporal information – Information about the task at hand, if appropriate.	• To provide the patient with information about his or her environment

NURSING DIAGNOSIS: ALTERED THOUGHT PROCESSES (*CONTINUED*)

Nursing Interventions *(continued)*	Rationales *(continued)*
• If your care plans include validation, engage the patient, using clues from the patient to accomplish your goals. For example: – If the patient wants to return home to care for children, say that a neighbor has agreed to take them to her house for the night. – If the patient refuses to eat because he or she can't pay for the meal, provide a canceled receipt or scrip the patient can use in payment.	• To avoid unduly stressing the patient without compromising your ability to communicate with him or her
• Assess the patient for signs of an underlying condition or disease, such as an infection or an adverse reaction to medications.	• To determine whether there is an underlying cause of the patient's altered thought processes and identify it
• Avoid arguing with the patient when he or she is experiencing a delusional episode.	• To avoid additional stress on the patient

COLLABORATIVE MANAGEMENT

Interventions	Rationales
• Consult with the psychiatric staff about the patient's condition.	• To determine what, if any, psychological problems underlie the patient's delirium or dementia
• Consult with the health care provider concerning the patient's medication regimen.	• To determine if the patient is suffering from an adverse drug reaction, causing the altered thought processes
• Encourage the patient (if possible) and the family and other caregivers to track delusional episodes. Keep a written behavioral log.	• To determine if any environmental factors are causing the delirium or dementia and to provide suggestions for effective interventions

NURSING DIAGNOSIS: ALTERED THOUGHT PROCESSES (CONTINUED)

OUTCOME:

- The patient will experience little or no adverse effects from the delirium or dementia.

EVALUATION CRITERIA:

- The patient remains free from injury resulting from his or her dementia or delirium.
- The patient displays evidence of adequate thought processes based on the initial assessment.

Patient Teaching

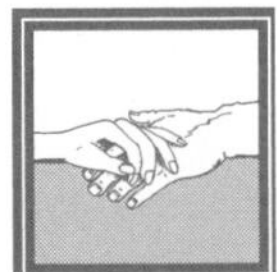

Patient teaching in cases of delirium or dementia is addressed to the patient and the family or other caregivers.

Depending on the severity of the patient's condition, it may only be possible to instruct the patient in the simplest of tasks. In every case, the patient should be included in self-care, socialization, and relaxation activities to his or her maximum capability.

Stress the ways to minimize hazards that can place a delusional patient at risk. Explain options such as the following:

- Provide a safe area to accommodate wandering behavior.
- Reduce environmental stimulation to eliminate additional stress on a patient's overtaxed abilities.
- Introduce devices to increase patient functionality, such as easy-to-handle table ware and easy-to-manipulate clothing.

Emphasize the importance of immediate assessment if the patient displays new or altered symptoms of dementia or delirium. Often the only sign of an underlying illness or infection is an alteration in the patient's behavior.

Documentation

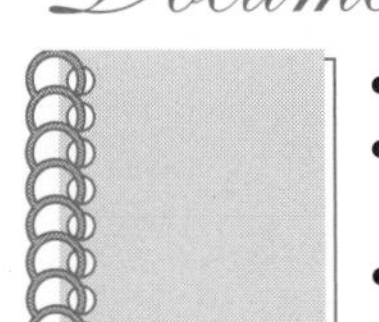

- Baseline vital signs and laboratory values
- Levels of cognitive abilities, communication skills, and perceptual skills
- Behavioral patterns, including causative factors, if identifiable, and effective interventions
- Medication requirements

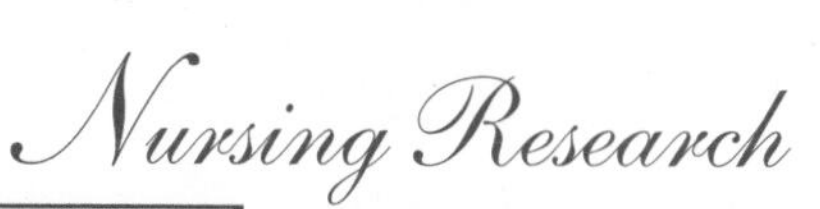

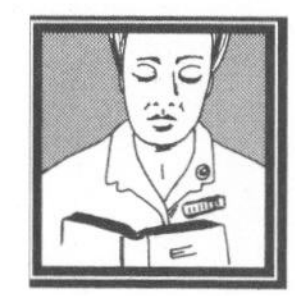

Delirium is commonly underrecognized and underreported in the geriatric population, although it is a serious factor in patient mortality. An estimated 70% of patients who become delirious are not identified as such by nurses or other health care providers and yet between 25% and 37% of patients who suffer delirium are dead within 1 month.

Foreman, M. "The Cognitive and Behavioral Nature of Acute Confusional States." *Scholarly Inquiry for Nursing Practice* 5, no. 1 (1991): 3–16.

Lipowski, Z. J. "Acute Confusion States in the Elderly." In *Critical Neurology of Aging,* edited by M. L. Albert. New York: Oxford University Press, 1994.

Chapter 9. Depression

▽ ▽ ▽ ▽ ▽ ▽ ▽

Introduction

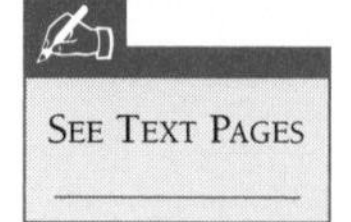

Depression is the most common psychiatric disorder suffered by elderly people. Between 15% and 25% of nursing home residents and about 15% of community-dwelling elders experience depression.

This same age-group, however, is the least likely to receive treatment. This is due to several factors, including the following:

- Underreporting by the patient because members of this age-group are the least likely to ask for help for psychiatric disorders
- Masking of depression symptoms by concomitant dementia, delirium, other medical conditions, or substance abuse
- Devaluation of the benefits of treatment for elderly people by health care providers

The primary goals of treatment and intervention include early recognition of the symptoms, prevention of recurring episodes, and mitigation of the effects of the current episode of depression.

Treatment options include behavioral strategies such as psychotherapy, pharmacologic interventions such as the use of antidepressants or sedatives, and electroconvulsive therapy (ECT), usually with patients for whom other options have failed.

Behavioral Strategies

Psychotherapy, especially when combined with medication, usually provides adequate relief from symptoms of depression. Therapy options include individual therapy for the patient, group therapy in which the patient can interact with others in similar situations, and family therapy in which the effects of the patient's depression can be addressed and alleviated for the whole family.

During therapy sessions, the patient and family or other caregivers can address issues such as the following:

- Patient self-esteem and feelings of worth or usefulness
- Patient feelings of fear and anxiety related to dependence, pain or illness, and loss of control
- Changes in the patient's role in the family
- Adaptation by the caregivers to the patient's demands brought on by illness or gradual decline
- Patient phobias or other specific conditions

Seeking help for depression is a major sign of the beginning of recovery.

Pharmacologic Interventions

Medication can provide significant relief from the symptoms of depression. As a general rule, antidepressants are the primary choice for medical intervention in depression.

Because the elderly patient is likely to be taking other medications, it's important to monitor the use of these drugs closely for adverse effects. Underlying illnesses or conditions may also alter the expected action of the medication.

Electroconvulsive Therapy

Electroconvulsive therapy is usually indicated for the depressed patient who does not respond favorably to psychological or pharmacologic treatment or for whom either of these techniques in contraindicated.

The success rate for ECT in the geriatric population is quite high; however, there is also a high relapse rate. Adverse effects are minimal, although older patients recover more slowly from the treatment and are more apt to suffer from post-ECT confusion than are younger patients. Close screening is necessary to rule out patients with underlying conditions that are contraindications for ECT.

Suicide Risk

Older people are more likely to commit suicide than younger people. In addition, suicide attempts by elderly people are more often fatal. It's vital to include an assessment of the patient's risk for suicide. Questioning the patient about suicidal thoughts or plans will not increase his or her risk for suicide. On the contrary, it will provide the information you need to make an early and more effective intervention.

NURSING DIAGNOSIS: ALTERED FAMILY PROCESSES

RELATED TO:

- *Patient's symptoms of depression, perceptual disturbances, or suicide risk*

Nursing Interventions	Rationales
• Assess the patient's relationship with other members of the family.	• To determine the organization of the family and better focus your interventions
• Discuss with the patient and the family characteristics of the new roles each will take.	• To support the patient in the changing situation
• Encourage open communication between all family members.	• To prevent misunderstandings and additional stress
• Provide information about the patient's illness or condition to the family, using the appropriate language.	• To facilitate their decision making
• Recommend that the family take advantage of counseling and other support services, as applicable.	• To reduce stress on the patient and family

COLLABORATIVE MANAGEMENT

Interventions	Rationales
• Consult with the psychiatric staff or social workers to discover other resources for the patient and his or her family.	• To provide additional options for the family to consider

OUTCOME:	EVALUATION CRITERIA:
• The patient and his or her family will report satisfaction with the new roles, whether they are temporary or permanent.	• The patient reports satisfaction with the arrangements that have been made.

NURSING DIAGNOSIS: ALTERED FAMILY PROCESSES *(CONTINUED)*

OUTCOME: (CONTINUED)

- The patient and his or her family will report satisfaction with the new roles, whether they are temporary or permanent. *(continued)*

EVALUATION CRITERIA: (CONTINUED)

- Obvious signs of disharmony, such as arguing, avoiding the patient, and noncompliance with arrangements, are reduced or absent.

NURSING DIAGNOSIS: ANXIETY

RELATED TO:

- *Coexisting depression, feelings of inadequacy, or inability to meet the demands posed by illness or other debilitating conditions*

Nursing Interventions	Rationales
• If there is an underlying illness or condition, explain the condition to the patient and family members or other caregivers, using appropriate language for the patient's level of understanding. Answer questions regarding surgical procedures, anatomy, body function, and psychiatric disorders.	• To ease unfamiliarity and discomfort and allow the patient some control over the situation
• Monitor the patient for signs of increasing distress, such as increased restlessness, difficulty sleeping, appetite changes, social withdrawal, and excessive crying.	• To provide an opportunity for early intervention
• Maintain a private, quiet environment. Encourage the patient to share concerns, and respond to each as appropriate. When listening, maintain eye contact and touch the patient in an appropriate and encouraging way.	• To maintain open lines of communication
• Promote a quiet environment by reducing external stimulation.	• To limit the drain on the patient's resources—mental, emotional, and physical

COLLABORATIVE MANAGEMENT

Interventions	Rationales
• Encourage the patient and family members to take advantage of counseling services and support groups, as appropriate.	• To develop effective coping skills
• Administer medications, as ordered: antianxiety drugs, sedatives.	• To decrease the patient's anxiety and fear

OUTCOME:	EVALUATION CRITERIA:
• The patient will appear calm and relaxed.	• Physical signs of distress, such as agitation, restlessness, and elevated respiratory rate, are decreased or absent.
	• The patient reports increased confidence, relaxation, and the ability to cope with anxiety.

NURSING DIAGNOSIS: CONSTIPATION

RELATED TO:

- *Medications administered to treat depression or patient's overall apathy toward eating, exercise, and other self-care behaviors*

Nursing Interventions	Rationales
• Monitor the patient's fluid intake and output closely. Encourage adequate fluid intake (1,500 to 2,000 mL daily).	• To assure adequate hydration
• Encourage the patient to eat well-balanced meals, including foods sufficiently high in dietary fiber.	• To decrease the risk of constipation
• Encourage the patient to participate in an exercise program.	• To decrease the risk of constipation and to promote the anxiety-reducing benefits of regular exercise

NURSING DIAGNOSIS: CONSTIPATION *(CONTINUED)*

COLLABORATIVE MANAGEMENT

Interventions	Rationales
• Consult with the health care provider concerning adverse effects of prescribed medications.	• To anticipate problems such as constipation and dry mouth
• Administer medications, as ordered: laxatives.	• To resolve constipation

OUTCOME:	EVALUATION CRITERIA:
• The patient will be free from symptoms of constipation.	• The patient's fluid intake and output are adequate.
	• Bowel movements are adequate and on a regular schedule.
	• Discomfort or abdominal pain is decreased or absent.
	• The patient reports resolution of his or her constipation.

NURSING DIAGNOSIS: HIGH RISK FOR VIOLENCE (SELF-DIRECTED)

RELATED TO:

- *Depression and suicidal intentions*

Nursing Interventions	Rationales
• Assess and treat the patient's immediate physical injuries, if he or she has inflicted any.	• To ensure patient safety
• Assess the patient's risk for suicide. Indications of high risk include the following: – Expression of thoughts of suicide – Plan for committing suicide – Possession of the means to accomplish suicide, such as a gun and ammunition or a supply of medication	• To identify the patient at high risk and focus your interventions on prevention

Nursing Interventions *(continued)*	Rationales *(continued)*
• Evaluate the patient's environment for items that the patient could use to harm himself or herself. Such items include the following: – Weapons, such as guns or knives – Razor blades or kitchen knives – Medications – Cleaning or gardening supplies	• To ensure patient safety
• Encourage the patient to describe the reasons behind the desire to commit suicide. If possible, clarify misconceptions that may be leading to suicidal thoughts.	• To promote open communication and ensure patient safety
• Encourage the patient to discuss his or her thoughts about suicide with you. Respond in a calm, non-judgmental way.	• To promote open communication and reduce the suicide risk
• If possible, establish an agreement with the patient such that he or she will not inflict harm or attempt suicide for a specific period of time. Continue to "renew" the contract while the risk of suicide is present.	• To allow the patient to develop effective coping methods and to encourage the patient to take responsibility for his or her own safety
• Monitor the patient following your facility's protocol for suicidal patients.	• To ensure patient safety
• Explain the patient's condition to his or her family and other caregivers, using appropriate language.	• To increase understanding
• Encourage the patient's family and other caregivers to involve the patient in pleasurable activities, according to the patient's interests and functional capacity.	• To distract the patient from suicidal thoughts and to promote patient safety

NURSING DIAGNOSIS: HIGH RISK FOR VIOLENCE (SELF-DIRECTED) *(CONTINUED)*

COLLABORATIVE MANAGEMENT

Interventions	Rationales
• Consult with the psychiatric staff concerning the patient's suicide risk. Refer the patient for evaluation and therapy.	• To ensure patient safety
• Administer medications, as ordered: antianxiety medications, antidepressants.	• To relieve the underlying anxiety and stress that may be causing the suicidal thoughts
• Consult with the health care provider to identify medications that might cause depression and lead to thoughts of suicide. Identify alternative medications.	• To reduce the role played by the adverse effects of the patient's medication
• Refer the patient to appropriate counseling and service agencies. Provide information about suicide hot lines and other emergency services.	• To ensure patient safety

OUTCOME:

- The patient will remain free from self-directed harm and no longer exhibit suicidal tendencies.

EVALUATION CRITERIA:

- The patient reports satisfaction with previously effective coping mechanisms and abandons plans for suicide.
- The patient's environment has been altered, if necessary, to prevent the patient from coming to harm.
- The patient's underlying depression is reduced through therapy, medication, or ECT, and subsequently, thoughts of suicide are no longer expressed.

NURSING DIAGNOSIS: HOPELESSNESS

RELATED TO:

- *Patient's condition or illness and exacerbated by depression*

Nursing Interventions	Rationales
• During all interactions with the patient, be sure to treat him or her with respect.	• To reduce the patient's feelings of hopelessness
• Encourage the patient to remember previous times when he or she successfully coped with anxiety or depression. Remind the patient of successes or triumphs, no matter how small.	• To focus the patient's attention on positive events and encourage the patient to use previously successful coping strategies
• Explain the goals the patient can anticipate happily, such as family visits, physical milestones, and successful treatments.	• To change the patient's outlook from one of negative anticipation to positive anticipation
• Listen actively to the patient as he or she explores "bad" feelings. Make it clear that everyone has these feelings at some time. Encourage the patient to identify the successful coping strategies of people he or she admires or respects.	• To develop rapport with your patient and encourage the patient to develop new coping strategies, based on the success of others

COLLABORATIVE MANAGEMENT

Interventions	Rationales
• Encourage the patient to take advantage of counseling or other social services.	• To increase the options available to the patient

OUTCOME:	EVALUATION CRITERIA:
• The patient will experience a reduction in feelings of hopelessness and exhibit a realistic understanding of his or her condition.	• The patient reports satisfaction with his or her method of coping with feelings of hopelessness.

NURSING DIAGNOSIS: HOPELESSNESS *(CONTINUED)*

OUTCOME: *(CONTINUED)*	EVALUATION CRITERIA: *(CONTINUED)*
• The patient will experience a reduction in feelings of hopelessness and exhibit a realistic understanding of his or her condition. *(continued)*	• A reduction in (or absence of) statements such as "What's the use?" and "Does anything make a difference?" occurs. • The patient participates in activities of daily living, self-care regimens, and social activities.

NURSING DIAGNOSIS: INEFFECTIVE INDIVIDUAL COPING

RELATED TO:

- *Patient's condition or illness or depression*

Nursing Interventions	Rationales
• Explore previously successful coping strategies with the patient.	• To help the patient use those strategies and develop new ones
• Encourage the patient to share his or her fears, concerns, or questions with you, the family or other caregivers, or other health care providers.	• To help the patient develop a support network
• Offer information about ways to increase the patient's ability to cope with changes in physical abilities or the effects of illness.	• To provide additional options for the patient to consider

COLLABORATIVE MANAGEMENT

Interventions	Rationales
• Consult with the physical or occupational therapy staff to discuss tools or other devices the patient can use to manage his or her changed circumstances.	• To provide additional options for the patient to consider

COLLABORATIVE MANAGEMENT *(CONTINUED)*

Interventions *(continued)*	Rationales *(continued)*
• Encourage the patient to consult with health care facility planners to determine what changes may need to be made if the patient will be entering a long-term care facility.	• To allow the patient to participate in planning his or her care
• Consult with the psychiatric staff to determine if underlying psychological disorders are altering the patient's coping mechanisms.	• To determine a course of intervention

OUTCOME:	EVALUATION CRITERIA:
• The patient will successfully cope with the effects of his or her illness, medical condition, or changing physical abilities and display few or no symptoms of depression.	• The patient reports satisfaction with coping behaviors.

NURSING DIAGNOSIS: SELF-ESTEEM DISTURBANCE

RELATED TO:

- *Patient's condition, illness, or changing capabilities or situation exacerbated by depression*

Nursing Interventions	Rationales
• Encourage the patient to explore feelings about his or her self-image—past, present, and future.	• To encourage the patient to understand that everyone experiences fluctuating feelings about themselves
• Provide activities for the patient that are appropriate for his or her interests and level of functional capacity.	• To increase the patient's satisfaction with his or her ability to complete the activities successfully

NURSING DIAGNOSIS: SELF-ESTEEM DISTURBANCE *(CONTINUED)*

Nursing Interventions *(continued)*	Rationales *(continued)*
• Educate the patient about methods for redirecting negative thoughts, such as guided imagery and meditation.	• To increase the patient's ability to cope with his or her situation

NURSE ALERT:
Note that some elderly patients might not be amenable to these interventions but may respond well to suggestions to think positive thoughts or to engage in prayer.

COLLABORATIVE MANAGEMENT

Interventions	Rationales
• Encourage the patient to take advantage of support groups or counseling, as appropriate.	• To provide the patient with additional outlets for improving his or her self-esteem
• Consult with the psychiatric staff about the patient's condition.	• To determine if underlying psychological conditions are contributing to the problem

OUTCOME:	EVALUATION CRITERIA:
• The patient will experience elevated self-esteem and realize his or her own worth.	• The patient reports satisfaction with his or her performance of self-care activities, social interaction, and so forth.
	• Evidence the patient cares for himself or herself adequately—a neat, well-groomed appearance—is apparent.
	• The patient actively engages in social interaction, as appropriate.

NURSING DIAGNOSIS: SELF-CARE DEFICIT (TOTAL)

RELATED TO:

- *Impairments in physical capability, perceptual disturbances or apathy caused by depression, and decreased communication skills*

Nursing Interventions	Rationales
• Concentrate on the patient's abilities to complete self-care tasks.	• To encourage the patient to do as much as possible for himself or herself
• Avoid completing the task yourself. Instead, assist or prompt the patient with touch or verbal cues.	• To decrease the patient's feeling of frustration and inadequacy
• Establish a routine for toileting activities, bathing, hair washing, and other self-care tasks.	• To decrease the patient's stress and anxiety over the self-care routines
• If a particular task is especially stressful for the patient, schedule it to take advantage of the patient's "good" time.	• To decrease stress on the patient
• Maintain a calm attitude toward the patient, respecting his or her privacy and dignity.	• To promote the patient's feeling of self-worth and confidence
• Compliment the patient on his or her grooming efforts.	• To increase patient compliance with care routine

COLLABORATIVE MANAGEMENT

Interventions	Rationales
• Consult with the physical or occupational therapy staff about tools or devices that can make self-care tasks easier for the patient, such as a long-handled brush for cleaning the back, a stool or chair for use in the shower, and a hand-held shower head.	• To provide options for the patient

NURSING DIAGNOSIS: SELF-CARE DEFICIT (TOTAL) *(CONTINUED)*

COLLABORATIVE MANAGEMENT *(CONTINUED)*

Interventions *(continued)*	Rationales *(continued)*
• Encourage the patient to dress in clothing that is easy to manipulate.	• To reduce the effort involved in self-care tasks
• Arrange for a hair dresser, dental hygienist, manicurist, or other technicians to help the patient maintain his or her appearance.	• To promote the patient's interest in self-care
• Consult with the health care provider about medications the patient is taking that might affect his or her appearance or hygiene requirements, such as hair loss from cancer treatments.	• To anticipate the need for special attention during self-care routines

OUTCOME:	EVALUATION CRITERIA:
• The patient will take as active a role as possible in his or her own care.	• The patient displays the ability to complete self-care tasks. • The patient presents a clean, neat, and well-groomed appearance.

NURSING DIAGNOSIS: SLEEP PATTERN DISTURBANCE

RELATED TO:

• *Depression*

Nursing Interventions	Rationales
• Assess the patient's current sleep patterns.	• To help identify problem areas
• Encourage the patient to regulate sleeping patterns by rising at the same time every day and getting the same amount of rest each night.	• To develop good sleeping habits and strengthen circadian rhythms
• Limit caffeine intake, restrict exercise or activity to the morning or early afternoon, and prepare for sleep with routine tasks.	• To reduce external causes for disturbed sleep

Nursing Interventions *(continued)*	Rationales *(continued)*
• Discourage the use of alcohol as a sleeping aid.	• To reduce the risk of establishing a fragmented sleep pattern in which the patient falls to sleep quickly but often awakes and finds it difficult to return to sleep
• Schedule nursing activities so that the patient can have an uninterrupted night's sleep.	• To encourage regular sleep patterns
• Provide a quiet, darkened room for sleep.	• To provide visual cues for the patient if he or she should awaken during the night
• Provide a nightlight in the patient's room.	• To orient the patient if he or she should awaken during the night
• If the patient does wake up during the night, determine if he or she needs to use the bathroom or is hungry, thirsty, or in pain and address those needs.	• To promote a return to restful sleep and to alleviate anxiety that may be caused by the patient's misperceptions of his or her environment

COLLABORATIVE MANAGEMENT

Interventions	Rationales
• Consult with other health care providers for suggestions to regulate the patient's sleep patterns.	• To develop a plan for coping with the altered sleep patterns
• Avoid medicines, unless necessary.	• To reduce the risk of injury if the patient does wake up and try to get out of bed unaided and to reduce confusion and restlessness that might be caused by an adverse effect of the medication

OUTCOME:	EVALUATION CRITERIA:
• The patient will experience restful, adequate sleep.	• The patient reports satisfaction with the amount of sleep and its quality. • Signs of excessive fatigue or hyperactivity are reduced or absent.

NURSING DIAGNOSIS: IMPAIRED SOCIAL INTERACTION

RELATED TO:

- *Changes in personality caused by depression*

Nursing Interventions	Rationales
• Encourage the patient to participate in as many activities as possible within the limits imposed by the patient's functional capacity.	• To reduce loneliness and increase interaction
• Engage the patient in normal conversation and interaction on a one-to-one basis as the opportunity presents itself.	• To encourage the patient to use his or her social skills
• Limit the amount of stimuli in the patient's environment.	• To avoid overstimulating the patient who is making tentative social contacts
• Focus the patient on a specific activity that is appropriate for his or her interests and functional capacity.	• To increase the patient's sense of self-worth and encourage involvement with others

COLLABORATIVE MANAGEMENT

Interventions	Rationales
• Consult with the occupational or physical therapists about activities in which the patient can participate with others.	• To encourage group involvement
• Encourage the patient's family or other caregivers to communicate with the patient frequently, either in person or over the phone.	• To decrease patient isolation
• Encourage staff members to include the patient in as many activities as possible.	• To encourage patient participation in social interaction

NURSING DIAGNOSIS: IMPAIRED SOCIAL INTERACTION (CONTINUED)

OUTCOME:

- The patient will enjoy social interaction with family, friends, other patients, and staff to the best of his or her abilities.

EVALUATION CRITERIA:

- The patient interacts successfully with others.
- Frustrated or stressed behaviors or catastrophic episodes are decreased or absent.

NURSING DIAGNOSIS: ALTERED NUTRITION (LESS THAN BODY REQUIREMENTS)

RELATED TO:

- *Depression or medications used to treat depression*

Nursing Interventions	Rationales
• Document the patient's weight, height, vital signs, and current nutritional status.	• To use as a baseline for evaluating patient status
• Monitor the patient's weight regularly—either daily or weekly—as the patient's condition warrants.	• To detect weight loss as quickly as possible
• Establish a consistent routine for mealtimes.	• To reduce patient confusion
• Identify techniques for increasing the likelihood that the patient will eat, such as preparing smaller, more frequent meals; preparing favorite foods often; and limiting the number of choices confronting the patient at mealtime.	• To increase patient compliance with the nutritional plan

COLLABORATIVE MANAGEMENT

Interventions	Rationales
• Consult with the dietitian to develop a diet plan for the patient.	• To ensure adequate nutrition

NURSING DIAGNOSIS: ALTERED NUTRITION (LESS THAN BODY REQUIREMENTS) *(CONTINUED)*

COLLABORATIVE MANAGEMENT *(CONTINUED)*

Interventions *(continued)*	Rationales *(continued)*
• Enlist the help of family members or other caregivers in making the dining experience pleasurable and comfortable for the patient.	• To promote patient compliance with the nutritional plan
• Monitor laboratory values, such as serum albumin and protein levels.	• To determine nutritional status and identify when supplements are needed
• Administer nutritional supplements, as ordered.	• To ensure adequate nutrition
• Consult with the health care provider to identify medications that might caused diminished appetite and suggest alternatives.	• To rule out medication as an underlying cause of malnutrition

OUTCOME:	EVALUATION CRITERIA:
• The patient will maintain optimum weight and adequate nutritional status.	• Weekly weight gain is in accordance with set goals. • Nutritional status is at appropriate levels for the patient.

NURSING DIAGNOSIS: ALTERED NUTRITION (MORE THAN BODY REQUIREMENTS)

RELATED TO:
- *Depression*

Nursing Interventions	Rationales
• Document the patient's weight, height, vital signs, and current nutritional status.	• To use as a baseline for evaluating progress

Nursing Interventions *(continued)*	Rationales *(continued)*
• Monitor the patient's weight regularly—either daily or weekly—as the patient's condition warrants.	• To detect weight gain as quickly as possible
• Encourage the patient to evaluate nutritional habits.	• To promote patient compliance and involvement
• Identify techniques the patient can use to decrease intake, such as eating low-calorie, low-fat snacks; eating smaller meals; and preparing low-calorie versions of favorite foods.	• To increase patient involvement
• Encourage the patient to explore the factors underlying the altered nutritional habits, if appropriate.	• To expand understanding of the disorder
• Explain the relation of stress, emotional disturbances, and other psychological factors to nutritional status.	• To increase the patient's understanding of the condition
• Establish goals for weight loss with the patient.	• To increase involvement in the self-care regimen

COLLABORATIVE MANAGEMENT

Interventions	Rationales
• Consult with the dietitian to develop a diet plan for the patient.	• To ensure adequate nutrition
• Obtain psychiatric counseling for the patient, if appropriate.	• To evaluate potential underlying disorders, such as bulimia or anorexia
• Consult with the physical or occupational therapy staff to develop an exercise plan for the patient.	• To promote weight loss and the anxiety-relieving properties of regular exercise

NURSING DIAGNOSIS: ALTERED NUTRITION (MORE THAN BODY REQUIREMENTS) *(CONTINUED)*

OUTCOME:

- The patient will make progress toward reaching and maintaining optimum weight.

EVALUATION CRITERIA:

- Weekly weight loss is in accordance with set goals.
- The patient reaches and maintains optimum weight.
- Nutritional status is at appropriate levels for the patient.
- The patient participates in a regular exercise program to the best of his or her functional capacity.

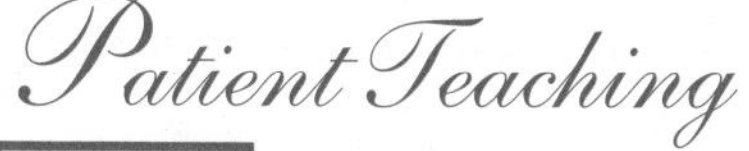

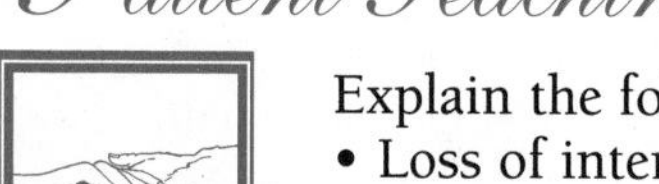

Explain the following signs and symptoms of depression:

- Loss of interest or enthusiasm in previously pleasurable activities
- Feelings of intense sadness, despair, irritability, or guilt
- Change in sleep patterns (increased or decreased)
- Unexplained change in weight or appetite
- Feelings of hopelessness or worthlessness
- Excessive fatigue
- Poor memory or inability to concentrate
- Unexplained physical problems, such as digestive difficulties, headaches, joint and muscle pain
- Altered sexuality patterns
- Thoughts of death or suicide

Explain options the patient has for treatment: counseling, medication, and ECT.

Stress that the use of alcohol or drugs will make the situation worse, providing only temporary relief. Keep in mind that although the general opinion is that elderly people are not at risk for substance abuse, it is actually a risk for this population and should be treated appropriately.

Identify the effects that the patient's medication or underlying illness or condition may have on depression symptoms.

Explain the risk factors and indicators for suicide. Risk factors do not eliminate a patient from consideration as a suicide risk; rather, they identify characteristics of the population most at risk. Indicators are evidence of the patient's inclination toward suicide.

Risk factors include the following:
- Middle- to upper-class white man
- Living alone with little social interaction
- Recent bereavement or relocation
- Chronic disease or pain
- Substance abuser, especially alcohol
- Previous suicide attempts

Indicators include the following:
- Expressions of powerlessness, hopelessness, excessive grief, or depression
- Suicide plan, including the means to carry out the plan, the location, and writing of a suicide note

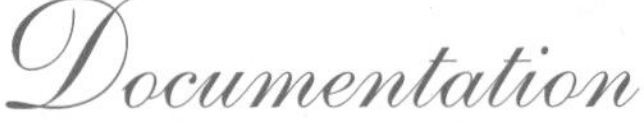

Documentation

- Medical history (to determine if an underlying disease or condition is causing or exacerbating depression symptoms)
- Mental status
- Nutritional and fluid intake status (older patients are especially vulnerable to dehydration)
- Compliance with care regimen

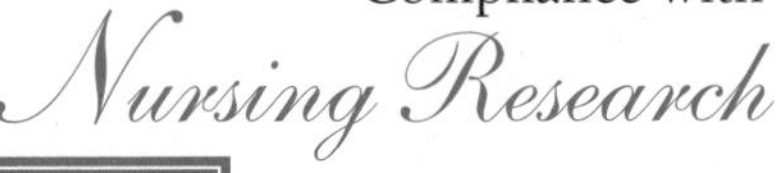

Nursing Research

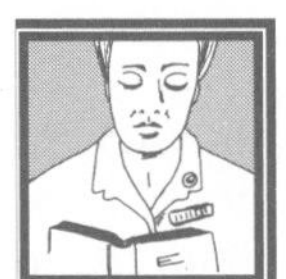

Your feelings and attitudes about aging and depression can alter the outcome of the patient's treatment. Patients are sensitive to your opinions about them and their condtions.

If you indicate that you think that the symptoms of aging are pathologic, rather than part of a natural progression, the patient may think that there is more wrong with him or her than there is. If you indicate that you believe that there is little benefit to treating depression in the face of other chronic disease, the patient will not get as much benefit from the treatment.

Regarding the suicidal patient, sometimes it is difficult to avoid feelings of anger toward the person who is trying to undermine your health care interventions. Again, your attitude is important in reinforcing the patient's feeling of self-worth and value.

Hogstel, Mildred O. *Nursing Care of the Older Adult*. 3rd ed. Albany, NY: Delmar Publishers, 1994, 204–233.

Chapter 10. Medication Problems

Introduction

Geriatric patients receive a large share of the prescription drugs that are dispensed. More than 25% of drugs dispensed are to patients aged 65 or older. The use and misuse of these drugs can pose serious risks to your patients. Many factors related to drug use should be considered for the geriatric patient.

Compliance Issues

There may be a great deal of variance between prescribed use and actual use. Patients may not understand the correct dosage requirements, such as amount, timing, or administration technique. They may also take matters into their own hands by adding a new medication, such as an over-the-counter preparation, or discontinuing a prescribed medication. Disagreement about the need or efficacy of a medication may also be a cause of noncompliance. Thorough and ongoing patient education is one way to address this issue.

Effects of Aging

As people age, they may react differently to medications from which they previously received benefits. There is also a wide variation in the effects of aging on the individual, so that what works well for one patient may be less effective for another patient of the same age. The following physiologic changes can cause unexpected responses to medication:

- Altered receptor sensitivity
- Diminished cardiac output
- Diminished hepatic blood flow
- Changes in the muscle-fat ratio
- Decreased kidney function
- Altered absorption, distribution, metabolism, and excretion of drugs caused by age-related changes, such as increased pH in the stomach and decreased motility in the GI tract

Another important change is in the time it takes for an adverse effect to develop. Such a reaction may take longer to develop in an elderly patient than in a younger patient. The reaction may even occur after the patient has stopped taking the medication.

Drug Interactions and Reactions

Many patients take a combination of drugs, both prescribed and over-the-counter, such as cold medications, sleeping aids, and vitamin supplements. Problems can arise in a variety of ways. Common interactions include the following:

- Drug-to-drug interaction. In this instance, two or more drugs the patient is taking lessen the efficacy of the drug or drugs; increase the potency of the drug or drugs; cause adverse reactions, such as delirium, GI problems, and alterations in the senses of vision, hearing, smell, taste, touch, or motion; affect blood chemistry results; and cause cardiovascular changes.
- Drug-to-disorder interaction. In this instance, the drugs the patient is taking to treat one complaint may exacerbate or cause another complaint or decrease the efficacy of medications taken to address another complaint.
- Drug-to-food interaction. In this instance, the drugs the patient is taking may cause reactions when the patient consumes his or her normal diet (or vice versa). The patient may experience food allergy-like reactions, a decrease or an increase in appetite, changes in intake resulting in weight loss or gain, or changes in the way the body uses nutrients. Certain foods may also alter the way the body absorbs and processes medications.
- Drug-to-environment interactions. In this instance, the effects of the drugs the patient is taking may be changed by exposure to elements in the patient's environment, or the patient may have to change his or her environment because of a drug's effects. For example, after taking certain drugs, the patient should limit sun exposure.

Discovering Adverse Reactions

Complicating the issue even more is the fact that the patient may not recognize or report adverse reactions. Some detective work on your part may be required to uncover such problems.

- The patient may be reluctant to admit to the problem because of embarrassment over the symptom or because of the fear of not being taken seriously.

- The patient may be unaware of the significance of the problem, thinking that the symptom is just a sign of aging and unrelated to medication.
- The patient may be unaware of the existence of the problem because other conditions mask or alter the symptom.

Adverse Reaction Reporting

If your patient experiences an adverse effect from one or more medications, you should report the episode, according to your facility's guidelines. This may include reporting to the Food and Drug Administration, depending on the medication involved and the severity of the adverse effect.

Your report should include the medication that is causing the adverse effect, a description of the effect, and a list of the interventions taken to address the problem. Note that you may need to consult with the health care provider or pharmacist to complete the report.

Patient Medication Evaluation

The evaluation of all patient medications is a vital element of health care for the geriatric patient. These evaluations should be conducted at the following times:

- During initial assessment
- When there is a change in the medication regimen
- When there is a change in the patient's condition, such as the diagnosis of a disease or the occurrence of an injury
- If the patient displays symptoms that appear to be unrelated to an existing or a known condition
- If the patient shows evidence of functional decline, such as an inability to complete activities of daily living
- If the patient displays worsening symptoms of an existing condition
- If the patient displays symptoms of delirium or worsening dementia

Routine, periodic assessments should also be done to ensure that the patient understands the use of each medication, that the medications are being used correctly, that they are not too old to be taken and are being stored properly, and that the patient has not added or removed any medications from the regimen.

Questions to Ask

The best method for performing a medication evaluation is to request that the patient or caregiver collect all medications and bring them to you for review. Examine each medication, one by one, and ask the following questions:

- What is the medication used for?
- When was it prescribed?
- What is the dose to be taken?
- What do you actually take?
- What are the adverse effects or warning signs and symptoms to report to the health care provider?
- Were there any special instructions about the medication, such as "Take with food"?

NURSING DIAGNOSIS: ALTERED HEALTH MAINTENANCE

RELATED TO:

- *Patient's lack of understanding or compliance with the medication regimen*

Nursing Interventions	Rationales
• Assess the patient's understanding of the health maintenance regimen and his or her current ability to successfully complete the required activities.	• To determine the areas on which to focus your interventions
• Explain, using language appropriate for the patient, what is required.	• To alleviate misunderstanding
• Encourage the patient, family, or other caregivers to take an active role in the health maintenance regimen.	• To encourage patient compliance
• Adapt self-care routines to take advantage of the patient's abilities and downplay his or her disabilities.	• To help maintain the patient's self-esteem

NURSING DIAGNOSIS: ALTERED HEALTH MAINTENANCE (CONTINUED)

COLLABORATIVE MANAGEMENT

Interventions	Rationales
• Consult with therapists, physicians, dietitians, and so forth to develop an effective plan for the patient to follow.	• To increase patient compliance

OUTCOME:	EVALUATION CRITERIA:
• The patient will take appropriate care of himself or herself and follow all recommended health maintenance requirements.	• The patient recovers from the disease or disorder or maintains an ongoing health status.
	• The patient participates in the planning of health care behaviors.

NURSING DIAGNOSIS: KNOWLEDGE DEFICIT

RELATED TO:

• *Medication regimen*

Nursing Interventions	Rationales
• Educate the patient about the prescribed medications, including purpose, dose, schedule, adverse effects, warning signs and symptoms, special instructions, and administration techniques.	• To increase the patient's understanding
• Encourage the patient to ask questions regarding the medications.	• To clarify the patient's understanding
• Assess the patient's readiness for learning. When he or she is ready for information, provide a variety of materials for review.	• To take advantage of the different ways people learn, such as by listening, seeing, and doing

Nursing Interventions *(continued)*	Rationales *(continued)*
• Include the patient's family and other caregivers in the educational program.	• To increase the likelihood that the patient will follow the self-care regimen

COLLABORATIVE MANAGEMENT

Interventions	Rationales
• Consult with other health care providers in stressing the importance of the health care regimen, especially the importance of using medications correctly.	• To ensure understanding of the importance of the health care regimen

OUTCOME:	EVALUATION CRITERIA:
• The patient will demonstrate adequate knowledge about his or her medication regimen.	• The patient can accurately describe the effects of the medication, its use and dosage, and any adverse effects and danger signs. • The patient complies with the medication regimen. • The patient seeks health care, if conditions indicate the need.

NURSING DIAGNOSIS: NONCOMPLIANCE

RELATED TO:

- *Lack of understanding about the medication regimen, cognitive or sensory impairments, or adverse effects of the medication*

Nursing Interventions	Rationales
• Assess the extent of the patient's noncompliance.	• To determine areas on which to focus your attention
• Explore the reasons for the patient's noncompliance, such as the following: – Misunderstanding of the instructions – Confusion or impaired mental processes	• To determine how to correct the noncompliant behavior

NURSING DIAGNOSIS: NONCOMPLIANCE *(CONTINUED)*

Nursing Interventions *(continued)*	Rationales *(continued)*
– Conflicting information from other sources – Cultural beliefs about the need or use of medications – Cost of treatments – Experience of adverse effects of the medication	
• If the noncompliance is related to misunderstanding or lack of knowledge about the care regimen, explain what is required, using language appropriate for the patient.	• To increase the patient's knowledge about the care regimen
• If the noncompliance is related to impaired mental processes, discuss the requirements with the patient's family or other caregivers.	• To increase the likelihood that the patient will receive the care he or she needs
• If the noncompliance is related to a sensory impairment, such as decreased vision, provide instructions written clearly in large print.	• To provide information in an accessible way

COLLABORATIVE MANAGEMENT

Interventions	Rationales
• If the noncompliance is related to the experience of adverse effects, discuss alternate medications with the health care provider.	• To resolve noncompliance related to adverse effects
• Encourage the patient to discuss his or her condition, instructions, care plans, or other aspects with appropriate members of your staff.	• To encourage the patient to make an informed decision about compliance

COLLABORATIVE MANAGEMENT *(CONTINUED)*

Interventions *(continued)*	Rationales *(continued)*
• Inform other staff members about the patient's decision as it affects them and their care activities.	• To avoid misunderstanding and confusion about the patient's desires

OUTCOME:	EVALUATION CRITERIA:
• The patient will comply with the care requirements as they have been agreed upon.	• The patient correctly identifies what is required to be in compliance with the medication regimen.
	• Evidence that the behaviors are being carried out, such as follow-up appointments being kept, improving condition, and completion of the full course of medication, is present.

NURSING DIAGNOSIS: SENSORY/PERCEPTUAL ALTERATIONS

RELATED TO:

- *Medication regimen*

Nursing Interventions	Rationales
• Assess the patient's sense of hearing, sight, touch, smell, taste, and motion.	• To determine the areas on which to focus your interventions
• Evaluate the patient's medications for adverse effects related to sensory perceptions.	• To identify medications that may be causing these effects and select alternative medications
• Assess the patient's ability to understand instructions concerning medications. Provide information in the form best suited to compensate for the patient's impaired sense or senses.	• To determine if sensory impairment is an underlying reason for noncompliance and identify alternatives for patient instruction

NURSING DIAGNOSIS: SENSORY/PERCEPTUAL ALTERATIONS (CONTINUED)

COLLABORATIVE MANAGEMENT

Interventions	Rationales
• Schedule an appointment with a vision or hearing specialist.	• To determine if corrective devices are needed
• If the sensory/perceptual alteration appears to be related to adverse effects of the medication, discuss alternate medications with the health care provider.	• To resolve underlying medication-related sensory/perceptual alterations
• Encourage the patient and family to take advantage of various support services for people with sensory impairment.	• To increase patient compliance with therapy designed to address sensory impairment

OUTCOME:	EVALUATION CRITERIA:
• The patient will experience a return to normal sensory perceptions.	• The patient reports restoration of the impaired sense. • The patient reports satisfaction with the corrective or assistive devices selected to compensate for sensory impairment. • The patient's medication has been changed, if appropriate, to one that does not cause sensory impairment.

NURSING DIAGNOSIS: ALTERED SEXUALITY PATTERNS

RELATED TO:

• *Medication regimen*

Nursing Interventions	Rationales
• Encourage the patient to discuss concerns with you.	• To alleviate the patient's embarrassment or worry that his or her concerns are insignificant or unimportant

Nursing Interventions *(continued)*	Rationales *(continued)*
• Educate the patient and partner, if appropriate, about the cause of the altered patterns of behavior.	• To increase the patient's understanding
• Stress the need to complete medical therapy to resolve the underlying condition, despite the adverse effect of altered sexuality.	• To maintain the patient's health status
• Encourage the patient and partner to share their concerns and thoughts and to develop other means of expressing affection and love.	• To provide options to the patient

COLLABORATIVE MANAGEMENT

Interventions	Rationales
• Consult with the health care provider to evaluate the patient for medical conditions that might be causing altered sexuality patterns.	• To rule out underlying medical reasons for altered sexuality patterns
• Discuss the patient's options with a sex therapist and the psychiatric staff.	• To develop more options for the patient
• Evaluate the patient's medications for adverse effects related to his or her sexuality.	• To identify medications that may be causing these effects and select alternative medications

OUTCOME:	EVALUATION CRITERIA:
• The patient will express satisfaction with sexuality patterns.	• The patient reports satisfaction with the return to normal patterns of sexuality or adjustment to new patterns.

NURSING DIAGNOSIS: SLEEP PATTERN DISTURBANCE

RELATED TO:

- *Medication regimen*

Nursing Interventions	Rationales
• Assess the patient's current sleep patterns.	• To help identify problem areas
• Evaluate the patient's medications for adverse effects related to sleep patterns.	• To identify medications that may be causing these effects and select alternative medications
• Discuss previous methods the patient has used to promote sleep.	• To encourage the use of successful coping methods and the development of new skills
• Encourage the patient to regulate sleep patterns by rising at the same time every day and getting the same amount of rest each night.	• To develop good sleeping habits and strengthen circadian rhythms
• Explain the effects of drugs and alcohol on sleeping patterns, and encourage the patient to avoid dependence on over-the-counter sleep aids.	• To promote the patient's natural sleep patterns
• Provide suggestions for altering activities, such as limiting caffeine intake, restricting exercise to the morning or early afternoon, and preparing for sleep with relaxation exercises or meditation.	• To provide the patient with options
• Encourage the patient to avoid daytime napping.	• To avoid further disruption of sleep patterns
• Schedule nursing activities so that the patient can have an uninterrupted night's sleep.	• To encourage regular sleep patterns

Nursing Interventions *(continued)*	Rationales *(continued)*
• Discuss the role played by diet and exercise.	• To minimize the effects of food, drink, and overexertion

COLLABORATIVE MANAGEMENT

Interventions	Rationales
• Consult with the psychiatric staff regarding patient counseling.	• To determine if there are underlying psychological causes for the altered sleep patterns
• Consult with the neurology staff regarding the patient's disturbed sleep patterns.	• To determine if there are underlying neurologic causes for the altered sleep patterns
• Consult with sleep specialists if the patient's altered sleep patterns are affecting activities of daily living.	• To develop a plan for coping with the altered sleep patterns
• Administer medications, as ordered: narcotics, sedatives.	• To promote restful sleep

NURSE ALERT:
Administration of medications to induce sleep should be considered as a last resort.

OUTCOME:	EVALUATION CRITERIA:
• The patient will experience restful, adequate sleep.	• The patient reports satisfaction with the amount of sleep and its quality. • Signs of excessive fatigue or hyperactivity are absent.

NURSING DIAGNOSIS: URINARY RETENTION

RELATED TO:

- *Effects of the medication regimen*

Nursing Interventions	Rationales
• Maintain the patient's micturition record, or teach the patient to record the information.	• To determine actual voiding patterns
• Evaluate the patient's medications for adverse effects related to urinary function.	• To identify medications that may be causing these effects and select alternative medications
• Monitor fluid intake and output.	• To ensure adequate hydration
• Encourage the patient to void at regular intervals.	• To encourage the development of a voiding schedule

COLLABORATIVE MANAGEMENT

Interventions	Rationales
• Review the patient's medications for those with the potential of causing anticholinergic effects.	• To identify alternate medications
• Consult with health care providers and, possibly, a urologist concerning the patient's condition.	• To determine if an underlying urologic condition may be causing incontinence, especially in relation to the patient's medications

OUTCOME:	EVALUATION CRITERIA:
• The patient will void the appropriate amount of urine.	• The patient's intake and output are relatively equal. • The patient takes in adequate fluid to support tissue hydration. • The patient voids an adequate amount each day.

ADVERSE EFFECTS OF MEDICATIONS

ADVERSE EFFECT	MEDICATIONS
Agitation	• Antidepressants • Antihistamines • Antipsychotics • Meperidine • Theophylline
Anemia	• Nonsteroidal anti-inflammatory drugs (NSAIDs)
Anorexia	• Digoxin
Anticholinergic effects	• Antidepressants • Antihistamines • Antipsychotics • Meperidine
Appetite changes	• Antianxiety drugs • Antihistamines • Antipsychotics • Ethanol (alcohol)
Aspiration	• Mineral oil laxative
Bleeding	• NSAIDs • Warfarin
Bruising	• Warfarin
CNS depression	• Antihypertensives • Benzodiazepines
CNS stimulation	• Caffeine

ADVERSE EFFECTS OF MEDICATIONS *(CONTINUED)*

ADVERSE EFFECT	MEDICATIONS
Cognitive impairment	• Benzodiazepines
Constipation	• Anticholinergics • Antidepressants • Antihistamines • Antipsychotics • Antisecretories • Codeine and derivatives • Iron supplements • Meperidine • NSAIDs • Tricyclic antidepressants • Verapamil
Delirium	• Anticonvulsants • Antidepressants • Anti-inflammatories • Antihistamines • Antihypertensives • Antiparkinsonians • Antisecretories • Bronchodilators • Codeine and derivatives • Narcotic analgesics • Neuroleptics • NSAIDs • Over-the-counter sedatives • Theophylline
Dementia	• Antisecretories • Benzodiazepines
Depression	• Antihypertensives • Antiparkinsonians • Beta blockers • Digoxin • Ethanol (alcohol) • Methyldopa

ADVERSE EFFECTS OF MEDICATIONS *(CONTINUED)*

ADVERSE EFFECT	MEDICATIONS
Depression *(continued)*	• Narcotic analgesics • Steroids
Diabetic control impairment	• Steroids • Nicotine
Diarrhea	• Alpha blockers • Antacids • Antiarrhythmic drugs • Anti-infectives • Beta blockers • Laxatives • Misoprostol
Diuretic effect	• Ethanol (alcohol) • Caffeine
Dry mouth	• Antidepressants • Antihistamines • Antihypertensives • Antipsychotics • Meperidine • Tricyclic antidepressants
Dystonias	• Metoclopramide
ECG changes	• Antidepressants • Caffeine • Digoxin
Edema	• Nifedipine
Excitation	• Antidepressants • Antihistamines • Antipsychotics

ADVERSE EFFECTS OF MEDICATIONS *(CONTINUED)*

ADVERSE EFFECT	MEDICATIONS
Excitation *(continued)*	• Meperidine • Theophylline
Extrapyramidal symptoms	• Antipsychotics
Falling, increased risk	• Analgesics • Antipsychotics • Benzodiazepines • Beta blockers • Narcotics • Sedatives
Fat-soluble vitamin malabsorption	• Mineral oil laxative
Fatigue	• Digoxin
Fluid retention	• NSAIDs • Steroids
Gait impairment	• Antidepressants • Antihistamines • Antipsychotics
GI bleeding	• Cholinergic blockers • Corticosteroids • NSAIDs • Quinidine
GI distress	• Meperidine
Headache	• NSAIDs • Steroids

ADVERSE EFFECTS OF MEDICATIONS *(CONTINUED)*

ADVERSE EFFECT	MEDICATIONS
Heart block	• Nitroglycerin
Hyperkalemia	• Beta blockers
Hypoglycemic response impairment	• Potassium-sparing diuretics • Potassium supplement
Hypotension	• Beta blockers
Incontinence	• Antihypertensives • Skeletal muscle relaxants
Infection	• Caffeine
Kidney function impairment	• Antibiotics • Steroids
Lethargy	• Aminoglycoside antibiotics • NSAIDs
Light-headedness	• Anticonvulsants • Beta blockers
Memory loss	• Quinidine
Nausea	• Benzodiazepines
Nightmares	• Digoxin
Orthostatic hypotension	• Antidepressants • Antihistamines • Antipsychotics • Diuretics

ADVERSE EFFECTS OF MEDICATIONS *(CONTINUED)*

ADVERSE EFFECT	MEDICATIONS
Orthostatic hypotension *(continued)*	• Meperidine • Nitroglycerin
Osteoporosis	• Heparin • Steroids
Ototoxicity	• Aminoglycoside antibiotics • Aspirin • Furosemide • Quinidine
Photosensitivity	• Psychoactive medications • Tetracycline
Priapism	• Trazodone
Psychiatric disorder	• Steroids
Sedation	• Anticonvulsants • Antidepressants • Antihypertensives • Antipsychotics • Benzodiazepines • Codeine and derivatives • Ethanol (alcohol) • Trazodone • Tricyclic antidepressants
Sexual dysfunction	• Antidepressants • Antihypertensives
Sleep disorder	• Benzodiazepines • Caffeine • Theophylline

ADVERSE EFFECTS OF MEDICATIONS (CONTINUED)

ADVERSE EFFECT	MEDICATIONS
Urine retention	• Anticholinergics • Antidepressants • Antihistamines • Antipsychotics • Antisecretories • Meperidine • Tricyclic antidepressants
Weight changes	• Digoxin • Steroids

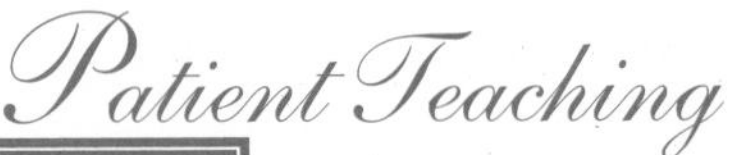

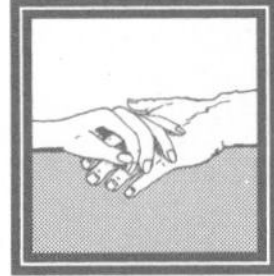

Explain to the patient, family, and other caregivers that it is important to understand all aspects of the medication regimen. This includes not only the purpose of each medication but also the relation between medications.

Emphasize that the medication regimen is one of the most important areas in which the patient and the health care provider must work as partners. The patient must follow the requirements accurately and not alter the regimen by discontinuing dosages or adding other medications without consulting the health care provider. The health care provider must take measures to ensure that each medication is necessary, is of sufficient dose to achieve the desired results but is not overprescribed, and is regularly evaluated for its effectiveness.

Identify in appropriate terms what adverse effects should be reported to the health care provider. Be especially careful to point out to other caregivers that worsening of existing conditions, such as dementia, is not necessarily the result of aging but can be the first sign of an adverse drug reaction.

Documentation

- Inventory of current medications
- Compliance with medication regimen
- Assessment of patient's understanding of the medication regimen
- Any adverse drug reaction experienced by the patient and the corresponding interventions

Chapter 11. Abuse

Introduction

Instances of abuse or neglect are often not reported or suspected, even when physical findings point to the problem. Estimates place the incidence of abuse or neglect at about 2 million cases annually nationwide.

Several factors can contribute to underreporting of abuse or neglect. They include the following:

- Fear of retribution causes many elderly people to be reluctant to report problems. Often dependent on their caregivers for food, shelter, and assistance, they may worry that they'll be left homeless.
- Societal attitudes that devalue the older adult may make some caregivers discount reports of neglect or abuse.
- Physical or mental impairment may prevent the older person from being aware of abuse or neglect or from communicating the problem to health care providers.
- Embarrassment over the situation can cause some elderly people to ignore or belittle the problem.

Mandatory Reporting

Many states require reporting of cases of suspected abuse. Both the patient who lives at home, either independently or in the home of his or her children or other caregiver, and the patient who lives in a care facility are at risk for abuse. In either case, your facility should provide guidance for the reporting of such abuse.

In 1987, Congress enacted substantial reforms regarding the treatment of patients in care facilities. Such patients have the right to be free from threats or actual abuse—either mental or physical—corporal punishment, discipline such as chemical or physical restraints, and involuntary isolation.

Types of Abuse or Neglect

In many cases, an elderly person may experience a combination of abuse and neglect. Some of the abuse and neglect is the result of willful activity, whereas some may occur because of ignorance on the part of the caregiver.

Physical abuse refers to a nonaccidental use of force. This includes physical assault, sexual assault, undue use of restraints, and punishment for perceived misdeeds.

Mental or psychological abuse refers to the infliction of mental distress and pain through the use of threats, intimidation, or abusive language.

Neglect refers to the withholding of care, including food, water, clothing, shelter, medications, appropriate hygiene, or health care. Neglect may result from willful actions or through inattention and ignorance.

Civil rights violation refers to the usurpation of an older citizen's legal rights, including access to his or her financial resources.

Self-inflicted abuse or neglect refers to actions by the patient that endanger himself or herself. This may take the form of self-directed violence or deliberate avoidance of health care behaviors.

Indicators of Abuse or Neglect

Evidence of neglect or abuse is the same for the geriatric patient as for other patients. If you suspect abuse, follow your facility's protocol for intervention and reporting.

Indications of abuse include the following:

- Injuries inconsistent with patient or caregiver report of the source or cause
- Multiple injuries in various stages of healing
- Bruises or lesions at ankle or wrist, indicating the use of restraints
- Bruises or scratches in the genital area
- Overall poor hygiene and grooming
- History of multiple health care providers and frequent emergency department visits
- Person accompanying the patient either dominates the conversation, answering for the patient, or is unaware of the reason for the patient's visit

- Unusual reactions to your questions or examination, such as flinching as if to avoid a blow
- Deterioration or worsening of an existing disease or disorder
- Increase in cognitive impairment
- Evidence of malnutrition or dehydration
- History of alcohol or drug abuse by the patient, family, or caregiver
- Evidence of caregiver stress

NURSING DIAGNOSIS: HIGH RISK FOR INJURY

RELATED TO:

- *Elder abuse*

Nursing Interventions	Rationales
• Assess the patient for evidence of physical abuse or neglect.	• To identify patients at risk
• Develop a supportive relationship with the patient, encouraging him or her to share concerns, fears, and worries. Listen in a nonjudgmental manner.	• To encourage the patient to identify abuse or neglect
• Reinforce the concept that everyone has a right to physical safety and adequate care.	• To support the patient in his or her decision to report the problem
• Encourage the patient to maintain as much control as possible over his or her activities. Suggest a buddy system or participation in group social activities.	• To reduce the potential for unreported abuse
• Assess the family or other caregiver for evidence of extreme stress and burnout or other risk factors that may contribute to abuse.	• To detect the potential for abuse before injury occurs
• Encourage the patient, family, and other caregivers to take advantage of support groups or other services, as appropriate.	• To reduce stress and provide assistance to the patient, family, and other caregivers

Nursing Interventions *(continued)*	Rationales *(continued)*
• If possible, establish a regular schedule for checking on the patient.	• To ensure patient safety

COLLABORATIVE MANAGEMENT

Interventions	Rationales
• Consult with the psychiatric staff, psychiatric nurse practitioner, or psychologists to schedule evaluation of the patient, family, and other caregivers.	• To determine if underlying psychological problems could result in abuse or neglect

OUTCOME:	EVALUATION CRITERIA:
• The patient will be free from injury, appear well groomed, and show no evidence of abuse or neglect.	• The patient does not report or show evidence of physical injury.

NURSING DIAGNOSIS: SOCIAL ISOLATION

RELATED TO:

- *Occurrence of abuse or neglect*

Nursing Interventions	Rationales
• Encourage the patient to participate in as many activities as possible.	• To reduce loneliness and increase interaction
• Engage the patient in normal conversation as the opportunity presents itself.	• To encourage the patient to use his or her social skills
• Focus the patient on a specific activity as appropriate for the patient's interests and functional capacity.	• To increase the patient's sense of self-worth and encourage involvement with others

NURSING DIAGNOSIS: SOCIAL ISOLATION *(CONTINUED)*

COLLABORATIVE MANAGEMENT

Interventions	Rationales
• Consult with occupational or physical therapists about activities in which the patient can participate with others.	• To encourage group involvement
• Encourage the patient's family or other caregivers to communicate with the patient frequently.	• To decrease patient isolation
• Encourage staff members to include the patient in as many activities as possible.	• To encourage patient participation in social interaction

OUTCOME:	EVALUATION CRITERIA:
• The patient will enjoy social interaction with family, friends, other patients, and staff to the best of his or her abilities.	• The patient interacts with others. • Frustrated or stressed behaviors are decreased or absent.

NURSING DIAGNOSIS: ANXIETY

RELATED TO:

- *Episodes of abuse or neglect*

Nursing Interventions	Rationales
• Encourage the patient to discuss fears, concerns, and questions with you. Explore specific areas about which the patient expresses anxiety, such as fear of abandonment or retribution.Emphasize that everyone has a right to personal safety and appropriate care.	• To ease anxiety and develop a relationship of trust with the patient
• Monitor the patient for signs of increasing distress.	• To prevent levels of anxiety and fear from becoming excessive

Nursing Interventions *(continued)*	Rationales *(continued)*
• Maintain a calm, relaxed demeanor, and reassure the patient that his or her concerns are appropriate and important.	• To reinforce the patient's confidence and alleviate anxiety over caregiver opinions about the patient's concerns
• Maintain a private environment. Encourage the patient to share his or her concerns, and respond to each as appropriate. When listening to the patient, maintain eye contact and touch the patient in an appropriate and encouraging way.	• To maintain open lines of communication

COLLABORATIVE MANAGEMENT

Interventions	Rationales
• Administer medications, as ordered: sedatives.	• To decrease the patient's anxiety and fear

NURSE ALERT:
Administration of medication should be considered a last resort.

Interventions	Rationales
• Encourage the patient and family members to take advantage of counseling services and support groups, as appropriate.	• To develop effective coping skills

OUTCOME:	EVALUATION CRITERIA:
• The patient will appear calm and relaxed.	• Physical signs of distress, such as agitation, restlessness, and elevated respiratory rate, are decreased or absent. • The patient reports increased confidence, relaxation, and the ability to cope with anxiety.

NURSING DIAGNOSIS: FEAR

RELATED TO:

- *Episodes of abuse or neglect, threat of violence or retribution, and emotional stress*

Nursing Interventions	Rationales
• Assess the potential for harm to the patient through either active abuse or neglect.	• To identify areas on which to focus your interventions
• Report suspected abuse, according to the protocol established by your facility. Inform the patient of measures taken to ensure his or her safety.	• To ensure patient safety
• Encourage the patient to develop a plan for dealing with the abusive situation, including the following: – Developing a buddy support system – Identifying other resources for care and help, such as hot lines and crisis prevention agencies – Making an escape plan	• To encourage the patient to take responsibility for his or her safety
• Encourage the patient to contact the appropriate counseling services.	• To increase knowledge and self-confidence to combat fear

COLLABORATIVE MANAGEMENT

Interventions	Rationales
• Refer the patient to social service workers, psychiatric staff, and other health care providers.	• To provide additional options for care to the patient
• Refer the patient and family to appropriate psychiatric counseling.	• To address the underlying causes of abuse

COLLABORATIVE MANAGEMENT *(CONTINUED)*

Interventions *(continued)*	Rationales *(continued)*
• Confer with legal authorities, patient representatives, and ombudsmen about the patient's legal position.	• To identify legal measures the patient can take to protect himself or herself

OUTCOME:	EVALUATION CRITERIA:
• The patient will no longer fear for his or her personal safety.	• The patient reports confidence in his or her personal safety.
	• Physical signs of fearful behavior, such as shying away from touch, excessive crying, or panic, are decreased or absent.

NURSING DIAGNOSIS: HIGH RISK FOR INFECTION

RELATED TO:

- *Bacterial or viral infection spread to the patient through assault or abuse or as a result of trauma from attack*

Nursing Interventions	Rationales
• Assess the patient for pre-existing disposition to infection, especially the status of his or her immune system.	• To prevent onset or worsening of infection
• Monitor vital signs for changes that indicate infection, such as elevated temperature and rapid heart rate.	• To prevent onset or worsening of infection

NURSE ALERT:

In the elderly patient, symptoms of infection may not be clear-cut. For example, your patient might not exhibit a true temperature spike (101.5°F [38.6°C]) but still have an infection. Similarly, the patient using beta blockers will not demonstrate tachycardia.

NURSING DIAGNOSIS: HIGH RISK FOR INFECTION *(CONTINUED)*

Nursing Interventions *(continued)*	Rationales *(continued)*
• Encourage the patient to drink fluids, maintain adequate nutrition, and rest frequently.	• To prevent onset or worsening of infection
• Record the events of the assault accurately, and document all injuries.	• To determine the patient's risk of infection.
• In the case of sexual abuse, obtain a thorough sexual, gynecologic, menstrual, and contraceptive history. Evaluate pregnancy status, if appropriate.	• To identify factors to rule out as risks of infection

COLLABORATIVE MANAGEMENT

Interventions	Rationales
• Obtain complete blood count with erythrocyte sedimentation rate.	• To determine the presence of infection

NURSE ALERT:
The atypical presentation of symptoms of infection in an elderly person may lead to an inaccurate diagnosis of infection. For example, the patient's complete blood count may be only slightly elevated because the elderly person may be unable to mount a significant leukocytosis, or the erythrocyte sedimentation rate may be elevated because of the presence of chronic inflammatory diseases.

COLLABORATIVE MANAGEMENT *(CONTINUED)*

Interventions *(continued)*	Rationales *(continued)*
• Consult with health care providers to determine necessary diagnostic tests and evaluation procedures, such as the following: – Gonorrhea cultures – Chlamydia cultures – Spermatozoa cultures – Acid phosphatase – Protein-specific antigens – DNA typing – Vaginal cultures – Herpes simplex virus, hepatitis B, human immunodeficiency virus, cytomegalovirus – Vaginal wet mount	• To collect evidence and rule out specific infections
• Document and report all necessary information, according to your facility's protocol and state regulations.	• To meet the legal mandate and protect the patient's rights
• Administer medications, as ordered: antibiotics, antivirals	• To reduce or eliminate infection

OUTCOME:	EVALUATION CRITERIA:
• The patient will be free of signs of infection.	• Vital signs are normal. • Cultures and laboratory tests show no sign of infection.

NURSING DIAGNOSIS: SELF-ESTEEM DISTURBANCE

RELATED TO:
• *Experience of abuse or neglect*

Nursing Interventions	Rationales
• Encourage the patient to explore feelings about his or her self-image—past, present, and future.	• To encourage the patient to understand that everyone experiences fluctuating feelings about themselves

NURSING DIAGNOSIS: SELF-ESTEEM DISTURBANCE *(CONTINUED)*

Nursing Interventions *(continued)*	Rationales *(continued)*
• Provide activities for the patient that are appropriate for his or her interests and level of functional capacity.	• To increase the patient's satisfaction with his or her ability to complete the activities successfully
• Educate the patient about methods for redirecting negative thoughts, such as guided imagery and meditation.	• To increase the patient's ability to cope with his or her situation

COLLABORATIVE MANAGEMENT

Interventions	Rationales
• Encourage the patient to take advantage of support groups or counseling, as appropriate.	• To provide the patient with additional outlets for improving his or her self-esteem
• Consult with the psychiatric staff about the patient's condition.	• To determine if any underlying psychological conditions are contributing to the problem

OUTCOME:

- The patient will experience elevated self-esteem and realize his or her own worth.

EVALUATION CRITERIA:

- The patient reports satisfaction with his or her performance of self-care activities, social interaction, and so forth.
- Evidence that the patient cares for himself or herself adequately—a neat, well-groomed appearance—is apparent.
- The patient actively engages in social interaction, as appropriate.

Patient Teaching

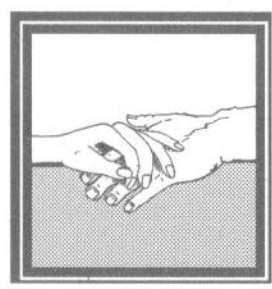

Educational efforts should include information provided to the patient about his or her right to safety and information to the caregiver about ways to cope with the tasks of caring for the patient.

Explain indicators and risk factors of patient abuse to the patient and caregivers. In this way, the patient understands that his or her health care provider will be aware of physical abuse. Caregivers will understand that their abusive actions will not go unnoticed or learn to recognize signs of abuse from other caregivers.

Indicators include the following:
- Bruises, cuts, scrapes, or other injuries at various stages of healing
- Multiple types of injuries, such as simultaneous puncture wounds and bruises
- Bruises or other injuries in unusual locations, such as the inside of the thigh
- Bruises or other marks that bear a resemblance to hand prints, hairbrushes, or rope burns, indicating a nonaccidental cause
- Signs of cowering, excessive timidity, or flinching when another person comes near
- Evidence of malnourishment or dehydration
- Explanation of injuries that is inconsistent with the actual injury
- Caregiver answering assessment and evaluation questions
- Person accompanying the patient has little or no information about the patient or the patient's condition
- Excessive passage of time between occurrence of an injury and seeking of treatment
- History of frequent emergency department visits or visits to multiple care facilities in an effort to avoid detection of a pattern

Risk factors include the following:
- Caregiver burnout
- Family history of abuse or neglect
- Substance abuse
- Dependency for financial support on caregiver
- Dependency for total physical care on caregiver
- Patient experiencing multiple pathologic conditions, such as dementia, chronic illness or disability, and total immobility

Documentation

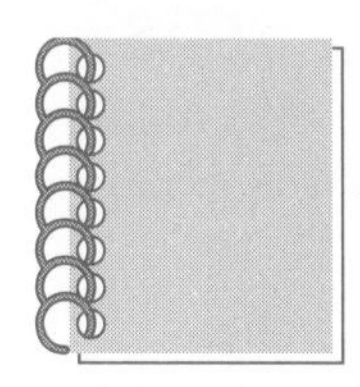

- Patient's physical condition, health history, and emotional status
- Evaluation of the risk of abuse or neglect
- Evaluation of the caregiver for risk factors
- Report to authorities, if applicable

NURSE ALERT:
When assessing a patient in a case where you suspect abuse, accurate documentation is crucial. It may be used in criminal prosecution. Be especially careful to note all relevant information about the patient's injuries or complaint, including the following:
- Patient's own words describing the injury or complaint
- Location, extent, healing status, number, and explanation of the injuries
- Results of diagnostics tests or procedures
- Interventions to address the injuries

If possible, photograph the injuries. Mark each photograph with the patient's name, the date, information about the injury, the names of the photographer and other health care professionals who examined the patient, and your name. The photographs should be retained as part of the patient's health history.

Chapter 12. Nutritional Concerns

Introduction

Changes in nutritional needs occur with aging. The following areas of concern exist for the geriatric patient and his or her caregivers:

- Meeting nutritional and care requirements for patients who can no longer ingest food by mouth and must be fed through parenteral or enteral routes
- Assisting the patient who can complete some of the tasks involved in eating but who may be experiencing problems related to dementia, overall weakness, illness, or a temporary change in condition
- Ensuring that the active patient receives adequate nutrition to meet his or her changing needs

Hazards of Malnutrition

Each of these patient groups presents challenges of its own. Underlying these concerns, however, is the fundamental goal of avoiding malnutrition. Malnutrition can cause many problems for your patient, including the following:

- Decreased energy
- Decreased immune response
- Decreased healing rate
- Decreased muscle tone
- Increased risk of tissue breakdown
- Increased fatigue
- Increased cognitive impairment

Nutritional Strategies

Strategies you can put into play will depend on your patient's individual needs. Perhaps the most important strategy is to recognize and remember that you are interacting with an individual whose tastes, food preferences, eating habits, and capabilities are unique.

The patient who requires enteral feeding must be assessed frequently to accomplish the following:

- Determine nutritional status.
- Avoid impairment of skin integrity.
- Prevent infection.
- Eliminate the risk of aspiration.

- Check the residual amount of food.
- Reduce diarrhea or constipation.

The following interventions are designed to help the patient who can complete some of the tasks involved in eating:

- Reduce the amount of ambient noise and activity.
- Provide verbal cues to remind the patient to swallow or drink fluids, for example.
- Eliminate clutter on the food tray, such as empty packaging and used bowls or plates.
- Serve favorite foods in small amounts at more frequent meals.
- Maintain a consistent routine at mealtimes, including using the same seat and location, having the same aide work with the patient, and providing food in familiar containers.
- Emphasize the importance of considering meals as activities to anticipate favorably, rather than as jobs to get done quickly.

Interventions for patients who are capable of managing their nutritional needs independently include the following:

- Educate about the correct balance of nutrients in the diet.
- Suggest ways to increase the appetite.
- Identify the correct weight, caloric intake, and nutritional status for the patient.
- Identify warning signs and symptoms related to diet and appetite that should be reported to the health care provider.

NURSING DIAGNOSIS: ALTERED NUTRITION (LESS THAN BODY REQUIREMENTS)

RELATED TO:

- *Poor appetite or lack of knowledge about proper nutrition*

Nursing Interventions	Rationales
• Document the patient's weight, height, vital signs, current nutritional status, and laboratory values, such as serum albumin and protein levels.	• To use as a baseline for evaluating progress
• Encourage the patient to evaluate nutritional habits.	• To promote patient compliance and involvement

Nursing Interventions *(continued)*	Rationales *(continued)*
• Explain dietary requirements, using the Food Guide Pyramid.	• To provide guidelines for the patient to follow

NURSE ALERT:
Note that many elderly patients may be unfamiliar with the Food Guide Pyramid or with the new food labeling standards.

• Identify techniques the patient can use to increase intake, such as eating high-calorie, high-protein snacks; eating smaller, more frequent meals; and preparing favorite foods often.	• To increase patient involvement
• Encourage the patient to explore the factors underlying altered nutritional habits, if appropriate.	• To expand understanding
• Explain the relation of stress, emotional disturbances, and other psychological factors to nutritional status.	• To increase the patient's understanding
• Establish goals for weight gain with the patient.	• To increase involvement in the self-care regimen

COLLABORATIVE MANAGEMENT

Interventions	Rationales
• Consult with the dietitian to develop a diet plan for the patient.	• To ensure adequate nutrition
• Obtain psychiatric counseling for the patient, if appropriate.	• To evaluate potential underlying disorders, such as depression and anorexia

NURSING DIAGNOSIS: ALTERED NUTRITION (LESS THAN BODY REQUIREMENTS) *(CONTINUED)*

COLLABORATIVE MANAGEMENT *(CONTINUED)*

Interventions *(continued)*	Rationales *(continued)*
• Administer nutritional supplements, as ordered.	• To ensure adequate nutrition

OUTCOME:	EVALUATION CRITERIA:
• The patient will make progress toward reaching and maintaining optimum weight.	• Weekly weight gain is in accordance with set goals. • The patient reaches and maintains optimum weight. • Nutritional status is at appropriate levels for the patient.

NURSING DIAGNOSIS: ALTERED NUTRITION (LESS THAN BODY REQUIREMENTS)

RELATED TO:

• *Chronic dementia*

Nursing Interventions	Rationales
• Document the patient's weight, height, vital signs, current nutritional status, and laboratory values, such as serum albumin and protein levels.	• To use as a baseline for evaluating progress
• Provide familiar elements at mealtimes, including using the same seat, having the same aide assist the patient, and using familiar plates, cups, and other utensils.	• To provide visual cues for the patient
• Reduce the environmental stimuli by turning off TVs, restricting visitors during mealtimes, completing mealtime activities in a calm and unhurried manner, and encouraging the patient to focus on the tasks involved in eating.	• To eliminate or reduce the effects of environmental press

Nursing Interventions *(continued)*	Rationales *(continued)*
• Provide finger foods or high-calorie snacks.	• To provide food in easy-to-manipulate forms
• Provide the minimum level of assistance required to help the patient complete the task. Assistance may involve the following: – Verbal cues, such as "It's time to eat your soup" – Physical cues, such as touching the patient's arm to remind him or her of the task at hand – Modeling the task, hand over hand, to reinforce the behavior – Completing the task entirely or asking him or her to complete as much of the task as possible	• To assure that the patient is adequately nourished while encouraging him or her to complete as much of the task as possible
• Use creative solutions to the patient's resistance to eating. For example, if the patient refuses food, return it to the kitchen and place it on another plate.	• To increase the likelihood that the patient will consume sufficient food
• Invite the patient to participate in preparing the meal or in activities such as table setting or simple serving duties.	• To increase the patient's involvement and cooperation
• Introduce additional opportunities for nutrition into the patient's daily routine, such as afternoon snack breaks and morning coffee breaks.	• To increase opportunities for the patient to eat

COLLABORATIVE MANAGEMENT

Interventions	Rationales
• Consult with the dietitian to develop a diet plan for the patient.	• To ensure adequate nutrition

NURSING DIAGNOSIS: ALTERED NUTRITION (LESS THAN BODY REQUIREMENTS) *(CONTINUED)*

COLLABORATIVE MANAGEMENT *(CONTINUED)*

Interventions *(continued)*	Rationales *(continued)*
• Consult with the physical or occupational therapy staff about devices that can make eating easier, such as wide-handled utensils, plate guards, and double-handled mugs.	• To provide additional options for the patient
• Administer nutritional supplements, as ordered.	• To ensure adequate nutrition

OUTCOME:	EVALUATION CRITERIA:
• The patient will ingest adequate amounts of food and maintain optimum weight.	• Weekly weight gain is in accordance with set goals. • The patient reaches and maintains optimum weight. • Nutritional status is at appropriate levels for the patient.

NURSING DIAGNOSIS: ALTERED NUTRITION (LESS THAN BODY REQUIREMENTS)

RELATED TO:
• *Inability to ingest sufficient nutrients by mouth*

Nursing Interventions	Rationales
• Document the patient's weight, height, vital signs, current nutritional status, and laboratory values, such as serum albumin and protein levels.	• To use as a baseline for evaluating progress
• Increase the nutritional content of foods in the patient's diet, using the following methods: – Add fortified milk to foods usually prepared with water.	• To provide additional nutrition without increasing the volume of food

Nursing Interventions *(continued)*	Rationales *(continued)*
– Eliminate the use of low-fat products and introduce extra fat into sauces, soups, gravies, and vegetable dishes by adding margarine. – Add fruit to foods such as cereal, ice cream dishes, and milk shakes. – Add nonfat dry milk to foods such as cream sauce, potatoes, puddings, eggs, and gravy. – Administer medications with juice or milk rather than with water.	
• Provide frequent opportunities for eating, and take advantage of the patient's "hungry time," usually at the beginning of the day.	• To increase the patient's intake
• Introduce additional opportunities for nutrition into the patient's daily routine, such as afternoon snack breaks and morning coffee breaks, or provide snacks when administering medications.	• To increase opportunities for the patient to eat

COLLABORATIVE MANAGEMENT

Interventions	Rationales
• Consult with the dietitian to develop a diet plan for the patient.	• To ensure adequate nutrition
• Administer nutritional supplements, as ordered.	• To ensure adequate nutrition

OUTCOME:	EVALUATION CRITERIA:
• The patient will ingest adequate amounts of food and maintain optimum weight.	• Weekly weight gain is in accordance with set goals. • The patient reaches and maintains optimum weight. • Nutritional status is at appropriate levels for the patient.

NURSING DIAGNOSIS: HIGH RISK FOR FLUID VOLUME DEFICIT

RELATED TO:

- *Chronic dementia*

Nursing Interventions	Rationales
• Monitor the patient's fluid intake and output.	• To determine patterns of intake and output to more easily identify variations
• Assess for other signs of fluid volume deficit, such as altered mental status, increased anxiety, increased heart rate, poor skin turgor, dehydrated mucous membranes, and hypotension.	• To assure early detection of fluid volume deficit
• Encourage the patient to drink adequate fluid (1,500 to 2,000 mL daily).	• To assure adequate hydration
• Remind the patient to drink at mealtimes. Use physical and verbal cues to draw the patient's attention to the drink accompanying the meal.	• To encourage adequate fluid intake
• Provide additional opportunities for drinking besides mealtimes, such as morning or afternoon juice breaks.	• To encourage adequate fluid intake
• Reduce the patient's intake of caffeinated beverages, such as coffee and soda.	• To reduce the diuretic effect

COLLABORATIVE MANAGEMENT

Interventions	Rationales
• Consult with the health care provider to identify medications that may cause diuretic effects.	• To ensure adequate hydration
• Administer a fluid transfusion, as ordered.	• To alleviate fluid volume deficit

NURSING DIAGNOSIS: HIGH RISK FOR FLUID VOLUME DEFICIT (CONTINUED)

OUTCOME:

- The patient will experience adequate fluid volume.

EVALUATION CRITERIA:

- Urine output is normal (>30 mL/hr.).
- Serum electrolyte levels are within normal limits.
- Vital signs are normal.

NURSING DIAGNOSIS: HIGH RISK FOR IMPAIRED SKIN INTEGRITY

RELATED TO:

- *Enteral feeding causing diarrhea and the placement of feeding tubes*

Nursing Interventions	Rationales
• Assess the patient's skin for color, turgor, temperature, and texture.	• To determine appropriate interventions
• Examine, clean, and retape tube sites on a regular schedule (minimum of once a day).	• To reduce the risk of skin breakdown
• Determine if the patient experiences an allergic reaction to surgical tape or other skin care products.	• To reduce the risk of an allergic response
• If the patient is using a tube that exits from the nose, the tube should be readjusted regularly to prevent the development of pressure ulcers at the site.	• To prevent infection and damage to the skin
• If the patient is experiencing diarrhea, be sure to assess perirectal skin regularly (at least twice a day).	• To reduce the risk of skin integrity breakdown

NURSING DIAGNOSIS: HIGH RISK FOR IMPAIRED SKIN INTEGRITY (CONTINUED)

Nursing Interventions *(continued)*	Rationales *(continued)*
• Explore possible causes of tube feeding–related diarrhea, such as the following: – Contamination of formula – Strength of formula – Speed of administration	• To minimize or eliminate these causes
• Clean the perirectal skin with perineal solution after each bowel movement.	• To remove stool residue and preserve the acid mantle of the skin
• Be sure the perirectal skin is dried thoroughly after each cleaning and a moisture barrier is applied.	• To prevent damage to the skin
• If skin breakdown occurs, clean the area carefully using sterile saline solution. Cover the area with appropriate dressings.	• To promote healing

COLLABORATIVE MANAGEMENT

Interventions	Rationales
• Administer medications, as ordered: analgesics, antibiotic ointments.	• To ease discomfort caused by skin irritation and to reduce the risk of infection
• Consult with the health care provider to determine if an adjustment in the type of enteral feeding is required.	• To ensure adequate nutrition

OUTCOME:	EVALUATION CRITERIA:
• The patient's skin will be warm, dry, and intact.	• The skin is normal in color, turgor, and temperature. • Signs of edema or erythema are absent.

Patient Teaching

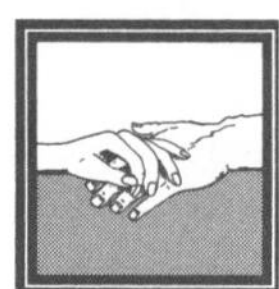

Nutritional guidelines form the basis for all patient teaching on diet, eating habits, weight loss and gain, and nutritional requirements.

Instruct the patient or caregivers in the basic requirements for adequate nutrition. Explain that each person may have specific requirements because of an underlying disease or disorder, such as a food allergy.

Provide information about making food and eating more attractive to those who have lost interest in mealtimes.

Explain nutritional goals to the patient or caregiver.

Emphasize that changes in weight, appetite, eating habits, or fluid intake may signal a serious condition that should be evaluated by the health care provider.

Documentation

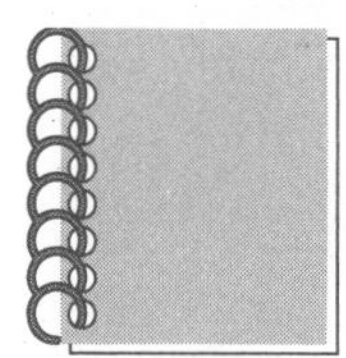

- Patient's weight (at admission and regular intervals)
- Caloric intake
- Fluid intake
- Eating patterns

Nursing Research

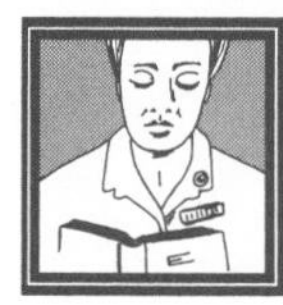

Nutritional studies identify four factors that influence a patient's intake: feeding technique, food consistency, time, and scheduling. By achieving the following goals in each of these categories, you can improve the results of your care planning and interventions.

- Feeding techniques should include appropriate use of verbal and physical cues, proper positioning of the patient, and consistent assistance.
- Food consistency must be adequate to the patient's needs.
- Adequate time must be allowed for patients to complete the tasks required for eating, with the appropriate

amount of assistance.
- Meals should be scheduled for times when the patient is most alert, least fatigued, and at his or her hungriest.

Osborn, Cheryl L., and Melody Marshall. "Promoting Mealtime Independence." *Geriatric Nursing* 13 (September-October 1992): 254–256.

Suggested Readings

Agency for Health Care and Policy Research. *Depression in Primary Care.* Rockville, MD: U.S. Department of Health and Human Services, April 1993.

Agency for Health Care and Policy Research. *Urinary Incontinence in Adults.* Rockville, MD: U.S. Department of Health and Human Services, March 1992.

Brady, Rebecca, Frances R. Chester, Linda L. Peirce, Judith P. Salter, Sharon Schreck, and Rosanne Radziewicz. "Geriatric Falls: Prevention Strategies for the Staff." *Journal of Gerontological Nursing* 19 (September 1993): 26–32.

Cole, Sandra L. "Dress for Success." *Geriatric Nursing* 13 (July-August 1992): 217–221.

Cooper, James W. "Preventing Falls and Fractures." *NH Practitioner* 2 (November-December 1994): 28–30.

Danner, Carol, Cornelia Beck, Patricia Heacock, and Tomye Modlin. "Cognitively Impaired Elders—Using Research Findings to Improve Nursing Care." *Journal of Gerontological Nursing* 19 (April 1993): 5–11.

Davidson-Johnson, Ilene. "Child and Elder Abuse Puts Patients and Physicians at Risk." *The Digest* 21 (Spring 1993): 1–4.

Duffy, Linda M. "Continence Management for the Frail Elderly and the Cognitively Impaired." *Urologic Nursing* 12 (June 1992): 66–68.

Faller, Nancy, and Katherine F. Jeter. "The ABCs of Product Selection." *Urologic Nursing* 12 (June 1992): 52–54.

Feil, Naomi. *The Validation Breakthrough.* Baltimore: Health Professions Press, Inc., 1993.

Fiers, Sheila. "Indwelling Catheters and Devices: Avoiding the Problems." *Urologic Nursing* 14 (September 1994): 141–144.

Gerdner, Linda A., and Kathleen Buckwalter. "A Nursing Challenge: Assessment and Management of Agitation in Alzheimer's Patients." *Journal of Gerontological Nursing* 20 (April 1994): 11–20.

Ginter, Sandra F., and Lorraine C. Mion. "Falls in the Nursing Home: Preventable or Inevitable?" *Journal of Gerontological Nursing* 18 (November 1992): 43–48.

Glickstein, Joan K., ed. "Urinary Incontinence: A Problem Not Often Assessed or Treated." *Focus on Geriatric Care and Rehabilitation* 3 (April 1990): 1–8.

Gross, Jan C. "Bladder Dysfunction After Stroke." *Urologic Nursing* 12 (June 1992): 55–63.

Jech, Arlene O. "Preventing Falls in the Elderly." *Geriatric Nursing* 13 (January-February 1992): 43–44.

Johnson, Patricia A., Marcia A. Stone, Anne M. Larson, and Cynthia A. Hromek. "Applying Nursing Diagnosis and Nursing Process to Activities of Daily Living and Mobility." *Geriatric Nursing* 13 (January-February 1992): 25–27.

Johnson, Vicki Y., and Mary A. Gary. "Urinary Incontinence: A Review." *Journal of the Wound, Ostomy and Continence Nurses Society* 22 (January 1995): 8–16.

Khan, Arifulla, Hugh Mirolo, Mary Helen Mirolo, and Dorcas J. Dobie. "Depression in the Elderly: A Treatable Disorder." *Geriatrics* 48 (June 1993): 14–17.

Kippenbrock, Thomas, and Mary E. Soja. "Preventing Falls in the Elderly: Interviewing Patients Who Have Fallen." *Geriatric Nursing* 14 (July-August 1993): 205–209.

Lachs, Mark S., Lisa Berkman, Terry Fulmer, and Ralph I. Horwitz. "A Prospective Community-Based Pilot Study of Risk Factors for the Investigation of Elder Mistreatment." *Journal of the American Geriatrics Society* 42 (February 1994): 169–173.

Marty-Nemeth, Pamela, and Kathleen Fitzgerald. "Clinical Considerations: Tube Feeding in the Elderly." *Journal of Gerontological Nursing* 18 (1992): 30–36.

McCormick, Kathleen A., Louis D. Burgio, Bernard T. Engel, Ann Schieve, and Eileen Leahy. "Urinary Incontinence: An Augmented Prompted Void Approach." *Journal of Gerontological Nursing* 18 (June 1992): 3–9.

McDowell, B. Joan, Sandra Engberg, Elizabeth Weber, Isabel Brodak, and Richard Engberg. "Successful Treatment Using Behavioral Interventions of Urinary Incontinence in Homebound Older Adults." *Geriatric Nursing* 15 (November-December): 303–307.

Mentes, Janet C. "A Nursing Protocol to Assess Causes of Delirium." *Journal of Gerontological Nursing* 21 (February 1995): 26–30.

Miller, Sue. "Polypharmacy." In *Decision Making in Gerontologic Nursing*, edited by P. A. Loftis and T. L. Glover, 72–79. St. Louis: Mosby, 1993.

Miller, Carol A. "Medications That May Cause Impairment in Older Adults." *Geriatric Nursing* 16 (January-February 1995): 47.

Nauss, Barbara H. "Abuse." In *Decision Making in Gerontologic Nursing*, edited by P. A. Loftis and T. L. Glover, 290–301. St. Louis: Mosby, 1993.

Osborn, Cheryl L., and Melody Marshall. "Promoting Mealtime Independence." *Geriatric Nursing* 13 (September-October 1992): 254–256.

Perkins, Karen R. "Depression." In *Decision Making in Gerontologic Nursing*, edited by P. A. Loftis and T. L. Glover, 282–285. St. Louis: Mosby, 1993.

Pillemer, Karl, and Beth Hudson. "A Model Abuse Prevention Program for Nursing Assistants." *The Gerontologist* 33 (1993): 128–131.

Plopper, Michael. "Common Psychiatric Disorders." In *Ambulatory Geriatric Care*, edited by T. T. Yoshikawa, E. L. Cobbs, and K. Brummel-Smith, 346–355. St. Louis: Mosby, 1993.

Rader, Joanne. “Modifying the Environment to Decrease Use of Restraints.” *Journal of Gerontological Nursing* 17 (1991): 9–13.

Richards-Hall, Geri. “Chronic Dementia: Challenges in Feeding a Patient.” *Journal of Gerontological Nursing* 20 (April 1994): 21–30.

Ryan, Judith W., Jane L. Dinkel, and Kerry Petrucci. “Near Falls Incidence—A Study of Older Adults in the Community.” *Journal of Gerontological Nursing* 19 (December 1993): 23–28.

Spier, Barbara E., and Martha Meis. “Maintenance Ambulation: Its Significance and the Role of Nursing.” *Geriatric Nursing* 15 (September-October): 277–281.

Sullivan, Gail M., and Lisa B. Korman. “Drug Associated Confusional States in Older Persons.” *Topics in Geriatric Rehabilitation* 8 (June 1993): 14–26.

Tappen, Ruth M. “Development of the Refined ADL Assessment Scale for Patients with Alzheimer's and Related Disorders.” *Journal of Gerontological Nursing* 20 (June 1994): 37–42.

Tarkowski, Linda. “Adverse Drug Reactions.” In *Decision Making in Gerontologic Nursing*, edited by P. A. Loftis and T. L. Glover, 68–69. St. Louis: Mosby, 1993.

Tarkowski, Linda. “Drug Interactions.” In *Decision Making in Gerontologic Nursing*, edited by P. A. Loftis and T. L. Glover, 70–71. St. Louis: Mosby, 1993.

VanOrt, Suzanne, and Linda Phillips. “Feeding Nursing Home Residents with Alzheimer's Disease.” *Geriatric Nursing* 13 (September-October 1992): 249–253.

Warkentin, Ruth. “Implementation of a Urinary Continence Program.” *Journal of Gerontological Nursing* 18 (1992): 31–36.

Wells, Thelma J. “Managing Incontinence Through Managing the Environment.” *Urologic Nursing* 12 (June 1992): 48–49.

Wood, Linda, and Glenda Cunningham. "Fall Risk Protocol and Nursing Care Plan." *Geriatric Nursing* 13 (July-August 1992): 205–206.

Wright, Barbara Ayn. "Weight Loss and Weight Gain in a Nursing Home: A Prospective Study." *Geriatric Nursing* 14 (May-June 1993): 156–159.

Yen, Peggy K. "Boosting Intake When Appetite is Poor." *Geriatric Nursing* 15 (September-October 1994): 284.

Yen, Peggy K. "Beyond the Basic Four." *Geriatric Nursing* 14 (March-April 1993): 109–110.

APPENDIX

LABORATORY VALUES IN THE ELDERLY

Because of a lack of research on the effects of aging and a lack of appropriate reference ranges for the elderly, there is still some controversy about a definitive list of "normal" lab values for older adults. Depending on which source you consult, you may find somewhat different information concerning individual tests. However, there is general agreement that there are certain values that do change with age, as well as some values that do not change. A summary of this information is included below. Please consult your facility's information for listings of normal adult ranges for various tests.

LABORATORY VALUES THAT DO CHANGE WITH AGE

VALUE	DEGREE OF CHANGE
Alkaline phosphatase	Increases by 20% between third and eighth decades
Biochemical tests	
Serum albumin	Slight decline
Uric acid	Slight increase
Total cholesterol	Increases by 30 to 40 mg/dL by age 55 in women and age 60 in men
HDL cholesterol	Increases by 30% in men; decreases 30% in women
Triglycerides	Increases by 30% in men and 50% in women
Serum B_{12}	Slight decrease
Serum magnesium	Decreases by 15% between third and eighth decades

LABORATORY VALUES THAT DO CHANGE WITH AGE *(CONTINUED)*

VALUE	DEGREE OF CHANGE
PaO_2	Decreases by 25% between third and eighth decades
Creatinine clearance	Decreases by 10 mL/min/1.73 m^2 per decade
Thyroid function tests	
T_3	Possible slight decrease
Thyroid-stimulating hormone	Possible slight increase
Glucose tolerance tests	
Fasting blood sugar	Minimal increase (within normal range)
1-hour postprandial blood sugar	Increases by 10 mg/dL per decade by age 30
2-hour postprandial blood sugar	Increases up to 100 plus age after age 40
White blood cell count	Decreases

LABORATORY VALUES THAT DO NOT CHANGE WITH AGE

Hepatic function tests

- Serum bilirubin
- Serum aspartate transaminase
- Serum alanine transaminase
- Gamma glutamyltransferase

Coagulation tests

Biochemical tests

- Serum electrolytes
- Total protein
- Calcium
- Phosphorus
- Serum folate

Arterial blood tests

- pH
- $PaCO_2$

Renal function tests

- Serum creatinine

Thyroid function tests

- T_4

Complete blood count

- Hematocrit
- Hemoglobin
- Red blood cell indices
- Platelet count

Source: Cavalieri, T. A., A. Chopra, and P. N. Bryman. "When Outside the Norm Is Normal: Interpreting Lab Data in the Aged." *Geriatrics* 47 (1992): 55–70.

NORMAL AGING CHANGES

The following chart reviews some major physical changes associated with the normal aging process and their nursing implications.

CHANGES	NURSING CONSIDERATIONS
Eyes	
Increased dryness	Patient may need prescription for eye drops and irritation
Increased light refraction	Use bright, indirect lighting; avoid glare (for example, shiny hospital floors).
Decreased accommodation	Avoid tasks requiring rapid accommodation.
Decreased color discrimination	Avoid tests requiring rapid accommodation or discrimination between colors in blue-green-violet spectrum (for example, reading a urine glucose strip).
Ears	
Sensorineural hearing loss Increased cerumen Decreased speech discrimination	Decrease or eliminate background noise; face patients when speaking to them; speak slowly; don't shout (it distorts speech); avoid high-pitched speech, particularly with S, Z, Ch, Sh sounds.
Taste/Smell	
Decreased or altered taste	Monitor for excessive use of salt and seasonings.
Decreased sense of smell	Patient living alone may be at high risk if unable to smell smoke or a gas leak.

NORMAL AGING CHANGES *(CONTINUED)*

CHANGES	NURSING CONSIDERATIONS
Taste/Smell *(continued)*	
Decreased protection of teeth and gums	More frequent mouth care; check for oral candidiasis; consider periodontal disease as a source of infection.
Heart	
Decreased response to stressors	Assess for evidence of poor response to stress.
Decreased cardiac output and heart rate at rest and with exercise	
Impaired function of baroreceptors	Incidence of postprandial hypotension is increased. Dangle patients' legs before getting them up.
Decreased sensitivity to antagonists	Response to drugs is altered.
Increased systolic pressure	Incidence of hypertension is increased.
Decreased number of cells in SA node	Irregular pulse is more common.
Increased systolic murmurs	N/A

NORMAL AGING CHANGES *(CONTINUED)*

CHANGES	NURSING CONSIDERATIONS
Lungs	
Increased residual volume	A "barrel chest" (A-P diameter) is a common assessment finding.
Increased chance of infection	Good pulmonary hygiene is especially important. Symptoms of pulmonary infections may present atypically; watch for lethargy, anorexia, confusion, poor functional ability. Promote increased fluid intake. Encourage meticulous mouth care to decrease aspiration of gram-negative bacteria.
Decreased ability to respond to increased oxygen demands	Pace activity with periods of rest.
Gastrointestinal	
Decreased protection of teeth, tongue, and gums from bacteria	Dental disease is not a normal consequence of aging. More frequent mouth care is required.
Decreased vitamin B_{12}, iron, folic acid, and vitamin D absorption	Patient may require supplementation.
Decreased protein digestion	Expect idiosyncratic drug reactions. Adequate nutrition is critical to maintain health status.

NORMAL AGING CHANGES *(CONTINUED)*

CHANGES	NURSING CONSIDERATIONS
Gastrointestinal *(continued)*	
Decreased gastric emptying	Patient may experience gastroesophageal reflux.
Decreased gastric hydrochloric acid production	Medication absorption may be affected if acidic medium is required.
Decreased glucose tolerance	Diabetes is more common.
Decreased hepatic protein synthesis	Expect idiosyncratic drug reactions due to decreased serum proteins.
Increased dysphagia	More than 3 swallows per mouthful indicates dysphagia.
Possible decrease in bowel motility	Constipation is not a normal consequence of aging. Monitor for signs of laxative abuse.
Renal	
Decreased blood filtration	Decreased renal function may account for drug reactions, such as increased half-life.
Possible decrease in glomerular filtration rate	Drugs competing for excretion sites can be a problem in polypharmacy. Creatinine clearance (not serum creatinine) should be used to calculate drug dosages.

NORMAL AGING CHANGES *(CONTINUED)*

CHANGES	NURSING CONSIDERATIONS
Renal *(continued)*	
Decreased bladder capacity	Incontinence is not part of normal aging.
Increased residual urine	Continence is critical in determining where a patient lives and how much support he or she needs.
Neurologic	
Loss of neurons, especially in cerebral cortex	Confusion is not part of normal aging and should be evaluated.
Decreased motor readiness, fine motor coordination, and balance	Risk of falls is increased. Prevention is critical.
Decrease in short-term memory and speed of processing information	Speak more slowly to allow time for information processing.
Impaired temperature regulation	Patient is more prone to hypothermia and hyperthermia; adjust room temperature appropriately.
Decreased reflexes, especially in lower extremities	Unilateral or focal signs are indicative of disease, not aging.
Sleep: Increase in total time in bed, increased wakefulness after sleep onset, increased sleep latency, decreased sleep efficiency	Avoid use of hypnotics and alcohol because they fragment sleep.

NORMAL AGING CHANGES *(CONTINUED)*

CHANGES	NURSING CONSIDERATIONS
Skin	
Thinning, drying, fragility of epidermis Decreased sebaceous activity	Prevention of trauma is key.
Decreased subcutaneous fat Decreased thermal sense	Pay attention to environmental temperature.
Decreased position and vibration senses	Don't get patients out of bed without proper footwear.
Decreased nail growth; thickening	Frequent podiatric care is required.
Musculoskeletal	
Increased incidence of fractures	Encourage mobility to prevent deconditioning. Teach fall prevention.
Osteoarthritis and osteoporosis are common	Regular weight-bearing exercise decreases bone loss. Reposition patients with joint disease every 1 to 2 hours.
Increased deconditioning (decreased lean muscle mass)	Encourage mobility to prevent deconditioning.

LIMITATIONS OF AGING AND ENVIRONMENTAL IMPACT

The following table reviews some potential limitations that the elderly may experience and the impact these limitations can have on the older adult's interactions with the environment. These limitations are not all normal consequences of aging; some represent pathologies.

LIMITATION	POTENTIAL ENVIRONMENTAL IMPACT
Age-related farsightedness: presbyopia	Reduced ability to focus on near objects.
Cornea less translucent; lets in less light	More external lighting is required to produce a clear image on the retina.
Sclera is less opaque and allows more light to enter the eye	More contrast is required because colors seem faded.
Lens of the eye may begin to yellow	Color vision becomes distorted, especially for shades of brown, blues, greens, and violets.
Pupil contracts and less light reaches the retina	Eyes are slower to accommodate when moving from lighted to dark room.
Cataracts cloud lens	Glare is more troublesome.
Macular degeneration	More magnification is required for vision.
Reduced field of vision	Peripheral vision narrows; may be slower to recognize environmental hazards.
Perceptive hearing loss	Normal sounds become distorted.
Requires hearing aid	Environmental sounds are amplified.

LIMITATIONS OF AGING AND ENVIRONMENTAL IMPACT *(CONTINUED)*

LIMITATION	POTENTIAL ENVIRONMENTAL IMPACT
Reduced sense of smell	Potentially dangerous odors (gas, smoke) are difficult to detect.
Sense of touch is less discriminating	Textures provide less stimulation.
Reduced body insulation and lower body temperature	Less tolerant of lower environmental temperatures.
Slower transfer of nerve impulses	Response to stimuli is slowed; reduced ability to regain balance.
Reduced strength and muscle tone	Difficulty getting up from a sitting position; tires more easily; shuffling gait.
Arthritic joints	Difficulty in climbing stairs and turning doorknobs.
Excessive need to urinate, especially at night	Need for an easily accessible bathroom.
Tires easily and is short of breath	Stairs and long hallways may be hard to manage.
Impaired short-term memory	May jeopardize safety by forgetting to turn off appliances.
Dizziness and hypotension caused by multiple medications	Higher risk of falling.

INDEX

D

E

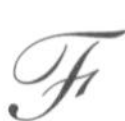

R

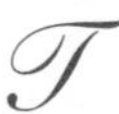

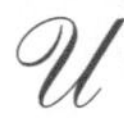

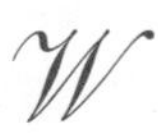

Order Other Titles In This Series!